Whose Child Is This?

Ethical, Legal, and
Theological Dangers
of "Surrogate Motherhood"

John Baycroft, editor

Anglican Book Centre
Toronto, Canada

1990
Anglican Book Centre
600 Jarvis Street
Toronto, Ontario
Canada M46 2J6

Copyright © 1990 Anglican Book Centre

All rights reserved. No part of this book may be reproduced, stored in a retrieval system, or transmitted, in any form or by any means, electronic, mechanical photocopying, recording, or otherwise, without the written permission of the Anglican Book Centre.

Typesetting by Jay Tee Graphics Ltd.

Canadian Cataloguing in Publication Data

Main entry under title:

Whose child is this? ethical, legal, social and
  theological dangers of "surrogate motherhood"

Includes bibliographical references.
ISBN 0-921846-28-2

1. Surrogate motherhood. 2. Anglican Church of Canada - Doctrines. I. Baycroft, John.
II. Anglican Church of Canada. General Synod.

HQ759.5.W46 1990   176   C90-094251-7

Contents

   Foreword

1. Introduction   *1*

2. The World of Surrogacy and Our Humanness   *4*
   Phyllis Creighton

3. Reflections on the Significance and Meaning of Surrogate Motherhood   *39*
   Marsha Hewitt

4. ''Rooted in Relation'': A Theological Reflection on Christian Values and Surrogacy   *55*
   Don Thompson

5. Surrogate Parenting - Legal Aspects   *80*
   Bruce Alton

6. Conclusions and Recommendations and Members of the Task Force   *93*

7. Response of Synod   *101*

8. Appendix   *104*
   Executive Summary of *Surrogate Parenting: Analysis and Recommendations for Public Policy,* The New York State Task Force on Life and the Law, May 1988

Foreword

It is an honour to be able to commend this report and the resolutions of the General Synod of the Anglican Church of Canada to the church and the community for study and action.

The authors of this report, members of the Task Force on Surrogate Motherhood of the Anglican Church of Canada, have made a significant contribution to a contemporary debate in this country. They have looked at the issue from both crucial points of view: first, in its broadest human setting, and second, in its deepest Christian implication.

The broad human setting requires an examination of technical, legal, historical and ethical considerations; the deep Christian implication requires a study of the scriptures and the tradition that has developed from them in the life of the Christian community. All this you will find in this report.

I know that this material is potentially significant for our society. What will make it actually significant is study and action by members of the church and others, and I pray sincerely that people everywhere will use this report for the purpose intended by the authors and by the General Synod of the Anglican Church of Canada.

Archbishop Michael G. Peers
Primate of the Anglican
Church of Canada

Introduction

Should Canadian society be allowed to change so that it becomes acceptable to buy babies and rent wombs? Is surrogate parenting consistent with Christian ethics? Are there any limits to the use of new technologies and social arrangements in response to human infertility? In the search for a social consensus on surrogacy the church is asked if it has any moral guidance to offer. Public policy and social values in a rapidly changing world adapt to new situations and possibilities. Unless individual believers and the churches participate in the discussion of ethical questions, the answers will probably be found without a Christian contribution.

In May 1987 the National Executive Council of the Anglican Church of Canada passed the following resolution:

> That this National Executive Council request that the Doctrine and Worship Committee examine the issue of surrogate motherhood with a view to providing the Anglican Church of Canada with research, information and guidance on this subject by the 1989 General Synod.

Subsequently, Bishop John Baycroft, as a member of the Doctrine Sub-Committee of the Doctrine and Worship Committee, was asked to chair a task force to implement this resolution. The primate suggested the names of Phyllis Creighton of Toronto and the Reverend Professor Bruce Alton of Trinity College, Toronto, and the Doctrine and Worship Committee approved the appointment of two additional members, Professor Marsha Hewitt also of Trinity College, Toronto, and the Reverend Doctor Don Thompson, Director of Studies at the Centre for Christian Studies in Toronto.

The task force held seven meetings. The first was a brief organizational one on 1 December 1987. We met three times in 1988, in January, May, and December, each time for two full working days. In 1989 we met four times for one day. Most of the work of the task force was therefore done privately by individual members. In the meetings we were able to reflect together on draft papers prepared by individual members and subsequently revised in the light of group discussion. We discussed some of the literature in the field. We were conscious that all of the members of the task force had read far more than time would permit us to discuss. However, fairly soon in our discussions we discovered that we had a common mind forming on the precise issue of surrogacy. This led us to try very hard to hold back from a judgment until we had listened to those who advocate surrogacy. For example, through conversing with an expert from a fertility clinic and by viewing video material documenting the dilemma of infertile couples, we understood the human pain involved in decisions about fertility. Yet it would have to be said that while this process led us to be sensitive to the need for loving pastoral support for couples who long for a child, nevertheless, the concern for couples made us more strongly opposed to the commercial exploitation of this human need and more outraged by aggressive campaigns to promote surrogacy.

It was important to review the conclusions about surrogate motherhood included in broader studies done elsewhere, for example in the Church of England,[1] in the Anglican Church of Australia,[2] and by the Congregation for the Doctrine of the Faith of the Roman Catholic Church.[3] We reviewed and generally approved the study of this subject by the Barreau du Québec.[4] Our conclusions are quite different from the majority view in the report of the Ontario Law Reform Commission.[5] We chose not to repeat the work done for General Synod and the Anglican Church of Canada by our Task Force on Human Life or by the National Executive Council's Committee on Human Sexuality. We did not consider it necessary to reproduce material from either *Artificial Insemination By Donor* by Phyllis Creighton, 1977,[6] or *A Study Resource on Human Sexuality* edited by James Reed, 1986.[7] We recommend both of these resource books published by the Anglican Book Centre, Toronto, Canada. The issue of artificial insemination by donor (AID), which is nowadays sometimes called therapeutic donor insemination (TDI) or semen donor insemination, is relevant to the achievement of a pregnancy in surrogacy arrangements.

To help those who wish to reflect on the issues surrounding surrogacy we offer a summary of our conclusions and recommendations and then some of the papers discussed by our task force.

Phyllis Creighton's paper helps us to know what is actually happening in Canada and the United States, and to assess the ethical concerns being raised. Marsha Hewitt analyzes the phenomenon from the perspective of a critical social ethics. Don Thompson uses biblical, liturgical, and canonical texts to identify the values in marriage and procreation which this practice would contradict, and therefore what is at stake theologically. Bruce Alton's paper shows that even in a situation which resembles a legal mine field, it is possible to make some clear legal and moral choices. We have received permission to reproduce as an appendix the executive summary from *Surrogate Parenting: Analysis and Recommendations for Public Policy* by the New York State Task Force on Life and the Law, May 1988, and we recommend also the rest of that report to those who are looking for a good summary of the discussion on surrogate parenting.

Notes

1. *Human Fertilisation and Embryology*, the response of the Board for Social Responsibility of the General Synod of the Church of England to the DHSS Report of the Committee of Inquiry, 1984, and *Personal Origins*, the report of a working party on human fertilisation and embryology of the Board for Social Responsibility, 1985.
2. Alan Nichols and Trevor Hogan, eds., *Making Babies: the Test Tube and Christian Ethics* (Canberra: Acorn Press, 1984).
3. *Instruction on Respect for Human Life in its Origin and on the Dignity of Procreation* (Rome: Congregation for the Doctrine of the Faith, February 22, 1987).
4. *Les enjeux éthiques et juridiques des nouvelles technologies de reproduction: le rapport du comité du barreau du Québec* (avril 1988).
5. Ontario Law Reform Commission, *Report on Human Artificial Reproduction and Related Matters*, 2 vols., 1985.
6. Phyllis Creighton, *Artificial Insemination by Donor: a Study of Ethics, Medicine, and Law in Our Technological Society* (Toronto: The Anglican Book Centre, 1977).
7. James Reed, ed., *A Study Resource on Human Sexuality: Approaches to Sexuality and Christian Theology* (Toronto: The Anglican Book Centre, 1986).

The World of Surrogacy and our Humanness

Phyllis Creighton

The Real World of Surrogacy

What's going on in surrogate motherhood? Why are some people enthusiastic about this practice so much in the news with the Baby M case? Why are others horrified — is it questionable? What do "experts" think about it, and in particular what do women say about it? How should we make up our minds about this approach to parenting? In the search for answers, this paper combines a historian's overview with ethical discussion of the issues. Behind it lie two concerns: does this approach to the creation of new life threaten to change how we think about procreation, about human relatedness, and even about our natures and destiny? What insight and response can the church offer that will help enhance our humanness?

Ours is a brave new world. Parenthood can be altered out of recognition. Recently we've seen a furor in South Africa when a 48-year-old grandmother bore her 25-year-old daughter's triplets created by *in vitro* fertilization,[1] and in Italy when a 20-year-old bore her 48-year-old mother's son, also created by IVF.[2]

There are now children born to women they are not genetically related to, and women who are genetically mothers but have never given birth. These are exotic versions of surrogate motherhood, which can give a child five parents, but usually only involves three. Surrogacy today is a social arrangement that by contract and reproductive technology — usually artificial insemination, rarely IVF — gets a woman to produce a man's child without sexual union with him. Fragmenting traditional marital conception, it separates pregnancy and childbearing from parental rights and responsibilities through an agreement to transfer the infant and maternal rights at birth from the birth mother — who is wrongly termed the surrogate — to the genetic father or, occasionally, the genetic parents.

Private arrangements of this kind were pioneered in 1976 by Noel Keane, a Michigan lawyer who, after five years of using volunteer surrogates (and five babies), began using paid ones and by September 1987 had achieved 177 surrogate births, while other agencies were multiplying in the United States.[3]

We learned of only a few such arrangements in Canada — cases of therapeutic necessity where life-threatening conditions ruled out pregnancy for a man's wife. Staff in several fertility clinics told us: "We don't do it, we don't know anyone who does it." One clinic source reported that physicians and staff overwhelmingly felt surrogacy should not be encouraged. We have heard doctors express moral qualms about surrogate motherhood as the sale of babies and the dehumanization of women, as well as concern about the psychological impact on the child and any other children of the surrogate mother. At the same time, some clinics make available to their clients material advertising the surrogate service at the Infertility Center in New York run by Keane, and he stated in May 1987 that at least 30 Canadian couples, mostly from the Toronto region, had used American surrogates.[4]

Philip Epstein, a Toronto lawyer experienced in this field, explains the process: typically a Canadian couple arranges for a woman to be inseminated in the United States, she comes to Canada for the birth, and an application is made to the courts to sever the ties between the surrogate and the child. He says:

> In all cases thus far, various judges of the Supreme Court of Ontario have approved that arrangement and made the various custody orders, which have then been followed by provincial court judges making the requisite adoption orders.

In the one publicized Ontario court case, which occurred in 1982, he observes: "The court did not engage [at that time] in any sort of discussion of the ethical, moral or legal principles involved in paying for a child."[5] Should the surrogate renege and refuse to surrender the child, however, he believes that Canadian courts will follow the example of English courts in rejecting such contracts.

When sociologist Margrit Eichler and researcher Phebe Poole investigated contract motherhood in the summer of 1988 for the Law Reform Commission of Canada they found it is going on to a limited but much greater extent than "experts" had estimated.[6] The 118 cases they turned up "represent a very conservative estimate which probably greatly underestimates the real extent of the phenomenon."[7] Most of the Canadian couples had hired U.S. women through U.S. agencies or employed a Canadian surrogate. Eleven American agencies had been involved, with Keane's having the greatest number of Canadian clients, but the researchers did not find any Canadian agency arranging contracts. Most cases entailed insemination of the birth mother with the sperm of the contracting husband. Some of the contractual mothers gave birth in a Canadian hospital using the name and health insurance number of the women to whom they planned to relinquish the baby. Are we, the public, already paying for this practice?

The data collected in the study substantiate the finding in earlier studies that the surrogate and her family usually are from a lower social and economic rung than the couple who hired her; they tended to have service or blue-collar jobs, and few had more than high-school education, while the couples seeking the babies tended to be in professional occupations. For Eichler and Poole, the high probability that a large amount of the activity is underground is the single biggest issue in contract motherhood.

Clearly surrogacy, with all its complexities, has arrived in Canada, so it is worth exploring. To understand what surrogacy is and what it means, the views of those for and against it need to be examined.

Lawyers Promoting Surrogacy

The surrogate mother, the book about Noel Keane, puts a strong plea for contract surrogate motherhood as a needed hope for anguished couples longing for children. Keane argues: how can anyone be against bringing a wanted baby into the world for a couple to love? The story told about Tom, his first client for a surrogate mother, is revealing. "The Lord intended women to have children" Tom says, "and I thought maybe one would want to do what came naturally and maybe help somebody else out while helping herself and her family." Implicit in Keane's approach are two reductionist notions: women are biologically made essentially for motherhood, and they are socially expected to be both self-giving nurturers and contributors to the economic well-being of the family. He sees himself as a pioneer in an altruistic movement. But he states that because of the hardship of pregnancy and childbirth few women will serve as surrogates for altruism and they must have money.

In Keane's legal-medical business, the child is the father's "investment" — anyway commercialization is the usual way in which individual needs are satisfied, he says. It is clear from the clients mentioned in the book that he arranges surrogacy contracts for people who already have children, and even for single men not intending to provide a social mother for the baby. "Every man has a right to reproduce himself," he believes. While this lawyer makes an appeal for reproductive freedom and the fulfilment of having children, his model is the commercial transaction.[8] The Baby M case has not changed his mind. For him, the lesson is that lawmakers must act to prevent similar cases in the future. Keane thinks jurisdictions not moving towards legitimating surrogacy are timid and tradition-bound, and he looks forward to the day when thousands of infertile couples will know the joy his couples have shared with him in the "surrogate birth of their child."[9]

U.S. law professor John A. Robertson, for whom surrogate motherhood is just another type of "collaborative reproduction" (added to artificial insemination by donor and adoption), approves of it as a free market model. He views it as a useful, needed service that a woman may offer for purchase, defining her as "not so much a substitute mother as a substitute spouse." The uncoerced exercise of economic choice is, apparently, its principal value. The purchaser of the service obtains the kind of child he or they want at their preferred time; the surrogate takes the job "primarily because the fee provides a better opportunity than alternative occupations" and in so doing makes a "considered, knowing choice."[10] Robertson sees difficulties arising from non-compliance with the contract and any psychological harms to the child as simply pains of the human condition that can be lessened by medical and legal services.

What arrangements do the lawyers propose for the business transaction of surrogate motherhood? The terms of the typical contract that lawyer Katie Brophy developed for use in her practice indicate that it is a deal securing a man's right to "his" child. The agreement signed by the surrogate and her husband is with the man whose inseminated semen will create her baby; it makes no mention whatever of any wife of his or any social mother. It sets out terms the surrogate must comply with in pregnancy (such as amniocentesis). It stipulates that she gets no compensation if she miscarries before the fifth month of pregnancy and only partial payment if she miscarries later, and that the full sum is to be paid her only when a child known by testing to be the natural father's is accepted by him.[11] The business deal is, then, for the sale of a child of approved quality? Do we want, for a social model, reproduction as quality manufacture?

Lori Andrews, a U.S. writer and lawyer long involved in studying reproductive issues, approves of surrogate motherhood, seeing it as medical treatment for the infertility of a wife (as well as, more rarely, for avoiding genetic risk). For her, childlessness is a particularly acute form of suffering — "infertility presents an unparalleled life crisis." Yet, oddly enough, she notes as a "drawback" of the programs run by the many firms founded mainly by lawyers that they make no medical check of the wife's reproductive system and so do not confirm her sterility. She also outlines, without criticism, cases of a single man's use of the arrangement to acquire a child. The surrogate motherhood she describes and accepts is, then, a wide-open business deal implementing complete reproductive freedom.

In explaining what motivates women to go through the nine months and birth of a contract baby, Andrews quotes Keane's psychiatrist Philip Parker: "Pregnancy is the last word in femininity." Apparently the reductionist notion of women colours her acceptance too. At the same time, the process she describes is designed to deny that the woman bearing the child is the mother. The contract she cites from Richard Levin of Kentucky Surrogate Parenting Associates stipulates that if the natural father dies, Levin is to get custody of the child until it is placed for adoption. Is the acquisition of male power over children through the sale of babies a key feature of surrogate motherhood under lawyers' aegis?[12]

Andrews is now promoting surrogacy as an inherent part of

reproductive freedom and choice for women. Although in her latest book, *Between strangers*, she makes it plain that agencies generally insist on anonymity and keep those making surrogacy arrangements from meeting each other, or formalize and discourage any contact, she touts a program being undertaken by William Handel's firm to encourage the contracting parties to develop an ongoing personal relationship with one another for a year. Her account portrays a humanized experience, and suggests that it helps the surrogate's self-growth, prompting new career and educational goals. Evidently to Andrews it seems a step forward that women can be more flexible and "don't have to feel absolutely 100 per cent attached to every child we carry." This apparent narcissism is described as expanding women's chances to become adventuresome and make a new contribution to society.

As for the critics, she hints, by lengthy theorizing from several psychologists, that surrogacy is disturbing because it demystifies the mythology surrounding motherhood, calls mother's love in question, and threatens those fearing abandonment or ambivalent about their own children — all without evidence. She seems to agree that public policy choices must ignore the wholeness of human experience, and any fears or "emotional taboos," in favour of a reason that seems curiously arid.[13] In any case Andrews believes in surrogate motherhood. She insists that "it will probably take Babies N, O and P before we get a law. . . . But eventually, I think that the law will allow surrogacy and regulate it."[14]

Laywers such as William Handel, of Surrogate Parent Foundation in California, criticize Keane's acceptance of all kinds of clients for babies (including fertile women), but only, they say, because they believe the most important thing right now is to get the concept of surrogate parenting into the law. Thus confining their clientele conservatively to stable married infertile couples, and showing this profile of the human needs to be met, plus the altruistic, girl-next-door surrogate,[15] is an essential strategy for political reasons, to avoid jeopardizing public sympathy.[16] But law professor Iwan Davies points out that reasons for surrogacy

> lie on a continuum between medical impairments which may be serious (for example risk to life) or minor (for example aggravating varicose veins) to . . . the great inconvenience

which pregnancy would entail (for example to career prospects). Any regulation of surrogacy would have to embrace the whole spectrum.[17]

Negative Legal Views

The New Jersey Supreme Court ruling on the Baby M case, issued on 3 February 1988, judges surrogacy harshly. Recognizing that the contract before it purports to provide a new way of bringing children into a family, the court observed that it inappropriately calls the natural mother the "surrogate mother." It invalidated the surrogacy contract (as conflicting with the state's law and public policy), and found "the payment of money to a 'surrogate' mother illegal, perhaps criminal."

Weighing the social parents' claim to be paying the surrogate only for services, the court said the arrangements amount to a private placement adoption for money. But the contract terms compared unfavourably with the protection provided in adoption: no clause allowing the natural mother to rescind her consent to surrender custody of the baby to its father, and a coerciveness (with money an inducement) depriving the woman of the time for careful decision-making that adoption provisions, with a mandatory delay after birth, ensure. The whole purpose and effect of the contract was to give the father the exclusive right to the child by destroying the rights of the mother. This, the court said, violates the state's public policy that the rights of the natural parents are equal. The harmful consequences appeared all too palpable. Thus the unanimous judgment held that:

> In New Jersey, the surrogate mother's agreement to sell her child is void. Its irrevocability infects the entire contract, as does the money that purports to buy it.

But the judges' strongest words cast a deeper doubt that surrogacy fits with human nature, given the bonding of mother to child. They averred that

> it is expecting something well beyond normal human capabilities, to suggest that this mother should have parted with her newly born infant without a struggle. Other than survival, what stronger force is there?

And they restored her rights as a natural mother neither unfit nor guilty of abandoning her child.[18]

George Annas, a U.S. lawyer-physician who teaches health law and writes for the American bioethics journal the *Hastings Center Report*, is a strong critic. "Surrogacy's essence is not science, but commerce," he says, and "commercial surrogacy promotes the exploitation of women and infertile couples, and the dehumanization of babies."[19] Treating infants like products or pets for the pleasure of adults, it devalues all children. As for the surrogates' claim to be making a noble gift, "she does not 'give' the baby away, she sells it." Furthermore the prime motivation behind surrogacy is neither the pain of infertile couples nor the right of women to enter into binding contracts, but rather "the broker's greed": "they are in business to make money."

Annas hails the final decision in the Baby M case for seeing through other deceptive claims: that surrogacy is family building, when it rests on destroying the mother-child bond, and that it involves new science and medical technology. The novelty is a reprehensible legal one — a contract drafted by lawyers to circumvent laws on custody, adoption, termination of parental rights, and baby-selling. He urges that the woman who gives birth should be identified as irrebuttably the child's legal mother, on two grounds. She contributes more to the child than the sperm donor or even an ovum donor, and the newborn needs an identifiable mother if decisions about its care have to be made quickly.

In his view, legislation is required to head off full surrogacy using IVF and transfer of an embryo not genetically related to the woman, for the gestational mother could be treated as an "incubator . . . with no rights or interests in the child at all."[20] He urges that the sale of children, and of human embryos, should be outlawed.

> Paying women to have children for other people is a bad idea; we should neither encourage it by law nor permit the power of the state, through the courts and the police, to be used to seize children from their mothers on the basis of preconception contracts.[21]

Ultimately, he warns, a social policy to prevent children from being seen as commodities that can be purchased and sold is essential, for otherwise we will be led to "a reconceptualization of human life and the value of human life."[22]

Reflecting on the legal and the human, Daniel Callahan, the philosopher who founded the Hastings Center, insists that the problems of the Baby M case — contending claims of mother and father that could have no mutually satisfactory outcome — are inherent in surrogacy. To avoid such disputes, we will have to cultivate women "willing to gestate and then give up their own children, especially if paid enough to do so," a trait we should not want to foster, even in the name of altruism. The issue should be decided at the social level: our society would be better off not having the complex difficulties surrogacy poses. The focus should be on the hard-headed concern underlying traditional worries about parenthood: "who is to be held accountable for the welfare of a child?" Surrogacy fails this test because it is a method of parenthood "built on confusion." And Callahan warns that, given the need to screen out women with the sensibilities of Mary Beth Whitehead (the mother of Baby M),

> we introduce as destructive a notion as can be imagined: a cadre of women whose prime virtue is what we now take to be a deep vice — the bearing of a child one does not want and is prepared not to love.[23]

Herbert Krimmel, a professor of law, goes further, arguing that it can never be ethical to conceive a human life in order to give it away. Recalling Nazi justifications for their medical experiments, he reminds us that

> to sanction the use and treatment of human beings as means to the achievement of other goals instead of as ends in themselves is to accept an ethic with a tragic past, and to establish a precedent with a dangerous future.[24]

Positive Reports on Surrogacy

The American Fertility Society
The 1986 report of the society's ethics committee is the major medical one favouring surrogacy, and since many Canadian doctors belong to the AFS, it needs analysis. The committee seemingly

analogizes surrogate motherhood to medical treatment for married couples. The inability of a woman to provide either the genetic or the gestational component for childbearing is given as the primary medical indication for use of a surrogate mother. They list as examples hysterectomy with removal of the ovaries, premature menopause, risk of passing on a genetic defect, inability to gestate due to severe hypertension, or a uterine malformation. Thus their treatment concepts encompass egg donation with the use of IVF. They do note that the extent to which surrogate programs "undertake an independent assessment of the infertility of the wife is unclear," and point out that drugs, surgery, or IVF might be suitable other options.

But they see surrogacy positively as possibly the only means to have a genetically related child, or "the only way in which [the husband] can conceive and rear a child with a biologic tie to himself." For them, it is also treatment for the non-existent child: it gives him or her "the opportunity to exist," and possibly to "be born into a much healthier climate than a child whose birth was unplanned," indeed, likely to a "rearing father [who] will have a greater sense of responsibility for the child than if the child were turned over to a stranger," as in the case of adoption. It is treatment for the surrogate mothers: "it offers them the chance to be altruistic"; moreover, "some surrogate mothers enjoy being pregnant," and, according to a study cited, about a third of them "may be using the process to help themselves psychologically" by seeking to relive the pregnancy experience satisfactorily, after having voluntarily aborted or having given up a child through adoption. Those doing it for a fee are "benefited by having another income option."

The committee does not recommend using a surrogate mother for the convenience of the rearing mother, because "nonmedical reasons seem inadequate to justify using a surrogate to undertake the risks of pregnancy and delivery." With all the benefits of the treatment foreseen, in the end even they express the need for appropriate data to resolve serious ethical reservations, and recommend that surrogate motherhood should only be "pursued as a clinical experiment."[25]

Since the report was issued a concern related to the safety of surrogacy has developed as a result of the spread of acquired immune deficiency syndrome (AIDS). In February 1988 the AFS issued revised guidelines for donor insemination stipulating that fresh semen should no longer be used and that all frozen specimens should be quarantined for 180 days and the donors retested to ensure they are free of the virus causing AIDS.[26] The Canadian Fertility and Andrology Society in October 1988 also advised its 347 members to use only frozen sperm and to quarantine it for at least six months and preferably up to one year for similar donor retesting.[27] Is the restriction being applied to the insemination of surrogate mothers? Nothing in the AFS journal indicates that special attention has been drawn to this application, though practitioners involved in surrogacy should be warned.

Unhappily, concern about AIDS is warranted: a surrogate mother, found only in pregnancy to be positive for the AIDS virus, has given birth to a baby with the same condition of whom neither she nor the contracting couple would take custody. The physicians who notified the *New England Journal of Medicine* of the case said: "We believe that both the semen donor and the potential surrogate mother should be screened for the presence of the HIV antibody" (the human immunodeficiency virus causing AIDS).[28] In connection with surrogate motherhood, the Canadian Medical Association has also issued a "warning of possible lawsuits by all the players, including the child, if the baby is born with an unforeseen handicap or is injured at birth."[29]

The Ontario Law Reform Commission
The OLRC's 1985 *Report on human artificial reproduction* is the only government-commissioned study that recommends the legitimation of surrogate motherhood. It was the work of five commissioners, all men, project director Bernard M. Dickens, and two male legal research officers. The commissioners think that a surrogate motherhood arrangement may be sought by a couple with an infertility problem that cannot be circumvented by other means — an abnormal or absent uterus, implantation difficulties, or chronic spontaneous abortion. They acknowledge that a fertile woman might want another woman to carry a child for her to avoid pregnancy, "possibly for reasons of career or vanity."

Since the scheme they recommend involves prior court approval of the arrangement and requires the prospective social parents to satisfy the court that they have a medical need which cannot be alleviated by other available means including the artificial conception technologies, it may seem that they analogize surrogate motherhood to medical treatment. But they also advise that for the initial period of regulation there should be no legislative provision to "address the question of such agreements made outside Ontario and intended for implementation in the Province." So broader reasons seem to be tacitly accepted, even though they recommend that participation in a surrogate motherhood arrangement known or believed to be intentionally evading the regulatory scheme should be subject to a fine.

In their scheme legislation is to provide for payment to the birth mother with the prior approval of the court. Isn't the OLRC's intent, then, to legitimize surrogate motherhood as a commercial transaction by contract? And the proposed contract is, by exception, to be irrevocable, unlike other commercial transactions. For when the child conceived under such an arrangement is born, the social parents are to be recognized as its parents for all legal purposes, the birth mother is to have no legal relationship to the child and is not to be named in the register of births, and even the fact that the child has been born to a surrogate mother is not to appear in the register.

What is being proposed is a legalized process for selection of breeders and purchasing parents by social agencies, physicians, and the courts, with paid, forced transfer of children. Specific enforcement of the contract means judicializing woman's power to procreate. It means transferring authority over the fruit of her body and thus over her body itself, first to the male whose semen creates her child, and secondarily to the legal system, which facilitates the arrangement and enforces the sheriff's right to seize the baby at the breast of a mother unwilling to surrender the newborn — as Mary Beth Whitehead and Baby M found out. It appears to recommend as progressive that we regard children as commodities which can be paid for — purchased, that is — by contract.[30]

The Barreau du Québec
The Quebec bar's April 1988 report was done by a committee of five lawyers — four of them women — appointed to study reproductive technologies. They see surrogate motherhood very differently from the OLRC. For them, surrogate motherhood entails risks far outweighing the benefits. They reject any paral-

lel between it and adoption, since surrogacy deliberately creates a situation which adoption simply seeks to remedy. Far from respecting human dignity, it treats the child as a marketable object. The infant, abandoned by its biological mother, is deprived of a bond of affection thought indispensable for sound development and faces the risk of devastating effects from revelation of the circumstances of its birth. Abandonment of an infant being an act generally condemned, they fail to see how, when planned and intended, it can be approved. As for the woman, in their view surrogacy reduces her body to an instrument and risks exploiting the needy. There is also no certainty that she can remain detached from the infant she carries and that she will not suffer a sense of guilt or inability to surrender the child, and thus the dreadful conflicts seen in the Baby M case.

In a wider sense, they think that surrogacy damages society by depersonalizing motherhood and upsetting family structures. The whole process trivializes the creation of life. The continuity of caring for the developing life is no longer maintained and pregnancy is reduced to a process of order by a couple, production by a female, and delivery. A variety of legal complexities concerning filiation also worried them. They therefore held that surrogate motherhood should be condemned from both ethical and legal viewpoints, surrogate contracts should be made unenforceable as contrary to public order, and medical or legal personnel or agencies facilitating such contracts should be subject to penal sanctions.[31]

The New York State Task Force on Life and the Law
A similar conclusion was reached by this group of 26 (9 of them women) drawn from the medical and legal professions and diverse religious bodies. Their May 1988 report, *Surrogate parenting*, canvasses social and ethical dimensions and public policy issues. They estimate that 750-1,000 babies have been born in the United States by surrogate contracts, through the help of 15 agencies, and they list Indiana, Kentucky, Louisiana, and Nebraska as states with laws declaring surrogate contracts unenforceable.[32] In their view, the Baby M case casts doubt on the idea that women applying to be surrogates are adequately evaluated, as well as on the likelihood that a standard of medical need for surrogacy could be defined and would be applied. They note that clinicians

who recruit surrogates claim that these women enjoy being pregnant and are motivated by altruism; but, on the basis of studies, they assert that the fee (usually $10,000) seems the major factor in the women's decision.

The task force argues that public policy recommendations must balance respect for individual freedom to make reproductive choices with upholding the social and moral values that form the "broadly shared vision of the public good." Surrogacy, in their view, is outside the scope of the basic right to reproduce, being neither a constitutional right nor a moral entitlement. The commercial nature of the arrangements, the potential conflicts between rights of the various parties, and the risks of harm all attenuate claims made to such reproductive freedom in the surrogate case. For them, surrogacy with fees and a contract to relinquish the child at birth is not in the best interests of children and threatens the dignity of women, children, and human reproduction. They see in "the fact that the practice condones the sale of children" a long-term potential for serious harm, for it represents a shift in "the way society thinks about and values children." The deliberate fragmenting of parenthood and of the family relationship prior to the child's conception poses high risks — court battles over custody, or abandonment of children born with anomalies. As for the claim made in the surrogate contract that any risks to the children are outweighed by the opportunity it gives them for life itself, they retort:

> the notion that children have an interest in being born prior to their conception and birth is not embraced in other public policies and should not be assumed in the debate on surrogate parenting.

In surrogate motherhood as a paid service they deplore the substitution of commercial values for the web of human meanings bound up with the bearing of babies. The service concept in itself depersonalizes women and devalues their reproductive role. And the assignment of market values, far from being an exaltation of "rights," is a derogation of the deeply human meanings bound up in procreation and maternal attachment. The birth mother bearing the child for income must deny the psychological dimensions of her experience and self. If she succeeds, self-alienation dehumanizes her; failure places her in the agony of conflict implicit in her attachment to the child. They see the transformation of gestation and human reproduction into commodities abstracted from family relationships, obligations, and caring, as especially problematic given advances in genetic engineering and thus potential new social and commercial options. For all these reasons they recommend that society should discourage the practice of surrogate parenting by legislation, declaring such contracts void, prohibiting payment of fees to surrogates, and barring surrogate brokers from operating.[33]

Canadian Legal Developments

In light of the coming trade deal with the United States (in place as of 1 January 1989), Sheila Copps in February 1988 introduced a private member's bill (C-284) in the House of Commons to prohibit a "rent-a-womb" market in Canada. Her intent was to make it a criminal offence (subject to a maximum two-year prison term) for any third party to initiate, solicit, or advertise for, or take part in surrogacy arrangements on a commercial basis. Both the Ontario and federal governments have been studying the broad questions related to reproduction and legislation. The federal speech from the throne on 3 April 1989 announced that a royal commission on reproductive technologies will be set up.

Women's Views

Feminist Gena Corea, who wrote *The mother machine*, says the issue in the new reproductive technologies, including surrogate motherhood, is not fertility, but rather the exploitation of women.[34] For her, the rationale Keane uses to justify the surrogate business stresses the partial element, the suffering of infertile couples, and obscures a clear vision of the actual social forces. Since the so-called surrogates are the actual mothers who allow themselves to be used for breeding, she terms them breeders. In her view, the business honestly analysed is trafficking in human beings, the child being treated as a commodity. Its underlying assumption is a throw-back to Aristotelian-Thomistic biology: woman is a vessel for man's seed.

Although it is often asserted that the infertile wife is the one benefiting, by the statements of Keane, Levin, and their clients "the overriding ethic is that the man's issue may be reproduced in the world." As for the claims that equality dictates women must be allowed to sell their eggs and wombs as men can sell their sperm, Corea agrees with feminist Andrea Dworkin's perception:

> Men have not yet grasped that women are not baby-making machines, and that women's bodies are not commodities best suitable to be sold. There seems to be no notion of personhood and integrity that applies a priori to women in men's minds. Otherwise it [surrogate motherhood] would be unthinkable.

For these feminists the social and economic construction of woman's will is in issue. By dint of low earnings and job ghettoes, a woman's economic status helps construct her "will" to sell her womb, as does her emotional structure — her overriding need to feel useful and wanted in a social system that affirms her as nurturer but in other respects accords women little value or opportunity for significant participation. The notion that selling the body is the highest expression of freedom, is, Dworkin observes, "a grotesque application of laissez-faire principles of capitalism."[35] Even more ominously, Corea reveals that the long-range goal of some agencies, John Stehura and the Bionetics Foundation, Inc., in particular, is to make surrogate motherhood more accessible by cutting the cost in half through the use of women in poverty-stricken parts of the U.S. and ultimately to one-tenth by using IVF, embryo transfer, and Third World women.[36]

In all this judicializing and commercializing, Corea thinks that motherhood is being dismembered and women devalued: "I'm not the mother, I only gave the egg"; "I'm not the mother, I only supplied the plumbing"; "I'm not the mother, just the incubator"; "I'm not the mother, I just provide care for the child." Their bodies are being treated by men as just receptacles — property. And to her it is significant that until less than a century ago throughout the world men by law could appropriate their children: the father had an absolute right to take the children away from his wife during marriage and fathers were routinely granted child custody in both England and America.[37]

Is Corea right that surrogate motherhood should be considered an upsurge in patriarchy? If she is right in seeing in the new reproductive technologies a meta-revolution, is surrogate motherhood altering the concept of humanness in ways diametrically opposite to Christian thinking about human dignity and wholeness?

Somer Brodrib of the Ontario Institute for Studies in Education, analyses the risks and issue in similar light in *Women and reproductive technologies*, a report done in 1988 for the federal department responsible for the status of women. What people see as the desperation of the infertile is shaping thinking and public policy. But in the midst of a changing definition of parenthood, the main concern — as shown in the OLRC report, she says — has been to assert men's ownership and paternity rights, not to attend to women's health or women's relationships to children or women's reproductive choice, an unjust inversion. Brodrib argues that surrogate-motherhood contracts "endanger the liberty and safety of women as a group, and are based on the economic inequality of women and the commodification of children."[38]

Suzanne R. Scorsone, the family life director of the Catholic archdiocese of Toronto, believes our humanity is on the line. The bond between child and mother is real, natural, and "essential to our survival as a society"; in exchanging it for money, as surrogacy does, the deeply human is reduced to the commercial. Thus surrogate mothers are selling a fundamental aspect of their humanity. In fact surrogacy, to her, is just a new name for concubinage, and the reintroduction of such exploitation is ironic in this age of women's rights. The surrogate, she notes, earns a pittance, while the lawyer as broker gets $10,000 for a few hours' work, at least $1,000 an hour on the deal, and the doctor $2,000 to $3,000. And "no matter how you cut it, surrogacy is baby-selling," she insists.[39]

Sidney Callahan, an American psychology professor, in discussing ethical guidelines for the use of alternative reproductive methods, takes a wide perspective. She stresses the role of marriage and family in securing the dignity and development of the generations. Since we are embodied creatures, she believes in the value of the cultural norms linking marital relationship, begetting, parenting, and extended kinship, which are based upon biological predispositions. She argues that if we legitimate the isolation of genetic, gestational, and social parentage and govern reproduction by contract and purchase, our culture will become even more fragmented, rootless, and alienated.[40]

Katha Pollitt, a writer who was pregnant with her own baby when the New Jersey lower court awarded Baby M to William Stern, scorns surrogacy. Of that court judgment she says:

> It seems that a woman can rent her womb . . . and get a check upon turning over the product to its father. This transaction is not baby selling (a crime), because a man has a "drive to procreate" that deserves the utmost respect, and in any case, the child is genetically half his. The woman he pays for help in fulfilling that drive, however, is only "performing a service" and thus has no comparable right to a child genetically half hers.

Surrogacy arrangements, she adds, "bear an uncanny resemblance to the all-sales-final style of a used-car lot." The patriarchal values of that court were matched by those of the contracts, which are "a way for men to get children." Since Mrs. Stern's name, like those of all the women in surrogate cases initiated by their husbands, was not on the contract, "rather than empower infertile women through an act of sisterly generosity, maternity contracts make one woman a baby machine and the other irrelevant." Stern's genes counted, and Mrs. Whitehead's genes, pregnancy, and childbirth together did not: "we might as well be back in the days when a woman was seen merely as a kind of human potting soil for a man's seed."[41]

Phyllis Chesler, an American psychologist who marshalled feminist support for Whitehead in the Baby M trial, sees surrogacy as "strip-mining the fertility of the poor." For her, the Baby M case is the quintessential custody battle which shows ours is "a culture that overvalues men, fathers, and money and undervalues women, mothers, and mother-child bonding." She queries whether denying their mutual bonding is a denial of an inalienable right and thus diminishes us all. From her considerable experience with interviewing and observing "contract mothers" she asserts that most "exhibit a remarkable degree of disassociation from their feelings, from their bodies, and from reality," as well as a fanatical naïvety and great pride in trusting and obeying. One surrogate profile she delineates is sobering —

> a *traditional* and *religious* woman who grew up in a rigorously *Christian household* where she was taught that a "good" woman is someone who sacrifices herself for others and transcends suffering by minimizing or denying it.

As for the prospects that the surrogate will get to enjoy a relationship with those who take her child, Chesler thinks most couples are grateful but "they also want nothing more to do with her after the baby is safely 'theirs'."[42]

Responses of the Churches

The Roman Catholic Church has taken a stand against surrogate motherhood. It insists that the suffering of spouses who cannot have a child must be properly evaluated. "The desire for a child is natural," but "the child is not an object to which one has a right: he is rather a gift." In Catholic understanding,

> the procreation of a new person, whereby the man and the woman collaborate with the power of the Creator, must be the fruit and the sign of the mutual self-giving of the spouses, of their love and of their fidelity.

Surrogate motherhood is not morally licit for the same reasons that artificial insemination by donor is not: *"it is contrary to the unity of marriage and to the dignity of the procreation of the human person."* The condemnation is thorough:

> Surrogate motherhood represents an objective failure to meet the obligations of maternal love, of conjugal fidelity and of responsible motherhood; it offends the dignity and the right of the child to be conceived, carried in the womb, brought in the world and brought up by his own parents; it sets up, to the detriment of families, a division between the physical, psychological and moral elements which constitute those families.[43]

Various Anglican bodies have expressed views on surrogacy. An American Episcopal Church committee reporting to the 1982 General Convention decried as narcissistic and self-indulgent the attitude that every individual has a right to a child as a form of self-fulfilment, and hence a claim on third-party assistance. Emphasizing that the surrogate mother must experience all the changes associated with child-bearing that will forge strong ties to the newborn, they urged the practice should be strongly condemned "as exploitative of the natural mother."[44]

The *Report on surrogate parenting and genetic engineering* submitted to the American Episcopal Church Convention in 1985 by its Standing Committee on Health and Human Affairs reiterated concerns about the mother's ties to the newborn "even though she is being treated as a childbearing vehicle by the recipient parents." They questioned whether her other children might not wonder, when the baby disappears, "Am I to be given away too?" They queried, as well, whether the adoptive parents could be comfortable knowing their happiness is tempered by the mother's sense of loss, and they also noted that the theology of their liturgy does not espouse the view that marriage cannot be fulfilled without a child. Thus a resolution was passed

> that the 68th General Convention, acting in the light of the Church's longstanding opposition to the selling of human sexual services, expresses its opposition to surrogate parenting for hire.[45]

In 1985, in *Personal origins*, a Church of England working party commented only on surrogacy through IVF, in which the birth mother is not the genetic mother. Viewing the process as a form of adoption, they hold that creating a child specifically for adoption is undesirable. And, especially where it involves the payment of money, they believe the practice is "undermining the dignity of women in the bearing of children they have no intention of mothering." Also, "strong bonding . . . takes place between a woman and the child she bears in her womb," and her potential unwillingness to let the child go after birth is a practical difficulty. They conclude that in surrogate motherhood the Christian institution of the family is fundamentally endangered, and thus that it cannot be morally acceptable as a practice for Christians.

The group backed the strong stand of the Warnock committee against surrogacy.[46] Since then, in February 1988 the General Synod formally supported the proposal of the British government "to leave all surrogacy arrangements outside the protection of the law."[47]

The Social Responsibilities Commission of the Australian Anglican Church has also rejected surrogate motherhood.[48]

How Shall We Decide?

Feelings
For many people, the deep longing of couples for a baby in their empty arms, and the radiant happiness they've seen in the handful of parents who have obtained a baby through surrogacy decide the question. The anguish of wanting a baby and not being able to have one makes us sensitive to the needs of the 10 to 15 per cent of women and men who do not succeed in procreating their own children. They tell us of the shock, the disbelief, the crushing blow to self-image and self-esteem that they suffer. We feel the pain in the cry: "What am I here on earth for? What will be left of me when I'm gone?"[49]

The emotional claim is heightened when in TV specials, in the press, on the radio, we hear healthy young women say they wanted nothing more than to do what was easy and fulfilling for them: to get pregnant and bear a child for a longing couple. The argument from human feelings and needs is powerful. And it has been promoted, to corner the market on feelings. Thus we have been helped to think that it is not right to deprive a couple of what many say is their only chance to have a child "of their own": surrogacy.

But whatever our sympathies, we must test the argument from feelings by reason. Surrogate parenting is now a business that makes big profits for brokers. We should not let them hide behind the grief of infertile couples. As Annas says, "They are not in business to help them" — if you don't have the $25,000 fee, no deal.[50] Note also that they take clients who have children of their own bodies but who cannot bear a child now by reason of age or a sterilization. Moreover, the power of feelings cuts several other ways. Surrogates have stressed their altruistic motives, their gladness at being able to make a pure gift of love. Some, indeed, say religious faith impelled them, because "the Bible orders us to do unto others as we would have them do unto us."[51] Others emphasize their satisfaction in being pregnant and claim that they needed this experience to complete their life.[52]

But a darker picture has begun to emerge. A counsellor who has worked, over five years, with 41 of them warns:

> Nearly all the surrogate mothers confessed that they had underestimated how difficult it would be to relinquish their babies. The symptoms of separation included uncontrollable sobbing, sleep dysfunction, aching arms, profound grief and the inability to look at any baby for several months without experiencing sharp, emotional pain.[53]

Consider the experience of Elizabeth Kane (a pseudonym). In 1980 on TV and in the press she spoke out passionately for surrogate motherhood as a generous loving gift to spare couples the anguish of infertility, the emptiness of their marriages. After the birth of the son she conceived for a couple by artificial insemination with the husband's sperm, she had a book written to tell about surrogacy as the fulfilment of her longing to help, a feeling so deep "it's part of my very soul." But *Birth mother*, the book she herself published in 1988, based on her diary, reveals her deepening dismay as the months of pregnancy wore on, as well as the painful impact of the surrogacy on her husband and three children. Able in public to deny her feelings, she told the media that she was just growing the baby for the man whose child it was, but when she had the ultrasound done at four months, she knew she loved the unborn one as much as her other children: "this child was mine!"[54]

Kane evidently was carried along by the reassurances of authority figures — her surrogate broker-physician and his legal team. She seems to have had little sense of her own self and little ability to look ahead. The realization that she would feel attached to this child for the rest of her life had not yet come home to her.

But the months after the birth and surrender of her child brought deep depression, contemplation of suicide, a damaged relationship with her husband, and deep disturbance in two of their children, with lasting consequences. Her reflections about her family are sobering. What she had meant to be

> a selfless act for an unknown family turned out to be a selfish act toward my own husband and children. . . . I had no idea my children would bond with their brother during the pregnancy or would spend years aching for the touch or sound of him.[55]

Over the years she had heard of other troubled surrogate mothers and children, and so she went to court for Mary Beth Whitehead and co-founded the Coalition Against Surrogacy. She now warns of unexpected long-term damage. Why? She has concluded that it is against human nature for a woman to psychologically disassociate herself from the child she is carrying. She also says, "I shudder to think of the loss of self-esteem when today's surrogate children are told they were bought and sold." What of the gift and the price? "I now believe that surrogate motherhood is nothing more than the transference of pain from one woman to another."[56]

Maternal Attachment and Bonding
Is the pregnant woman's bonding with her fetus — dismissed by the Ontario Law Reform Commission because of a dearth of "hard evidence" about its importance or extent,[57] but recognized by the New Jersey Supreme Court — a key consideration? Doctors, psychologists, and ethicists have long claimed that artificial insemination by donor is superior to adoption partly because pregnancy fosters the mother's attachment to her baby. So it seems that, with reproductive technologies, the argument from bonding is conveniently twisted either way. Women going through pregnancy share with their husbands and friends their growing awareness of the unique tiny life within them and their dawning affection for the unborn. Can it now in surrogacy seriously be claimed that prenatal bonding does not exist or matter?

But what about scientific evidence for such bonding? Study of the process is fairly new. Gale Bildfell Adam in her 1987 doctoral thesis on the subject (which was accepted at McMaster University) asserts:

> A review of the literature on maternal attitudes and feelings during pregnancy revealed substantial evidence that attachment to the unborn child develops well before the child is actually born.

In particular, studies of grief reactions following the death of newborns and of psychological difficulties after the birth of premature infants provided support for the view that maternal attachment develops during pregnancy. Her own research shows that during early pregnancy, women, whether pregnant for the first or a subsequent time,

> assign a sex and a personality to their unborn infants, visualize themselves and their infants in close physical contact following the birth and communicate with them verbally and by touch.

She found that women gain an increasingly clear image of the baby and that communication with the unborn is one area where maternal attachment increases as pregnancy advances.[58]

Couples going through the experience find York University psychiatrist Thomas R. Verny's book *Parenting your unborn child* useful. Drawing on knowledge gained in the past 30 years, Verny notes that the process of development makes the fetus by six months a feeling, sensing, aware, and remembering being. He points to research demonstrating that newborns recognize and prefer their mother's voice to that of another female or of their father.[59] Anthony J. DeCasper, the psychology professor he cites, has done a decade of research into fetal perception and memory. DeCasper says human responsiveness to sound begins in the third trimester of life, reaches sophisticated levels before birth, and fosters mother-infant bonding.[60]

In the book Verny wrote with John Kelly, *The secret life of the unborn child*, he explores the growing body of remarkable research in prenatal psychology, emphasizing that the unborn is shaped in personality by the nine months between conception and birth.[61] Drawing on research in Europe, Canada, and the United

States, he gives fascinating examples of the communication of a pregnant woman's emotions to her fetus and of their impact, with illustrations of serious consequences where they were negative. He sees pregnancy as the beginning of the meshing of mother-child rhythms and responses. Indeed, in his view, bonding between mother and unborn child is more beneficial than bonding after birth, and it is critical that they remain attuned to each other before the birth. Particularly important is the mother's love and respect for the life within her, a love and respect which, in the circumstances she has chosen, he questions whether a surrogate mother would allow herself.[62]

It has long been known that maternal emotions and, in particular, emotional stress, are transmitted to the unborn, both physiologically (through stress hormones) and psychologically (through behavioural communication).[63] Sensitivity and imagination tell us that a woman's refusal to become emotionally involved or to attach herself to the unborn life developing within her is a deprivation of warmth that may well affect it negatively. The ambivalence, anxiety, or dawning sense of the difficulty coming in the surrender after birth could be communicated to her fetus. These potential troubling experiences are not to be trivialized. But they pale before the painful wrench facing the newborn, who through nine months has known only his mother's ways and voice.

The evidence backs common observation and women's sense of the mutuality between mother and fetus. It is hardly surprising that these realities have served as cautious warning to thoughtful observers about the risks in surrogate motherhood. David Roy, who heads the Montreal Center for Bioethics, says the fact that the surrogate infant "is crudely and rudely ripped away from the warmth and sounds of the mother may have implications for the future development of the child."[64]

The knowledge being gleaned about attachment provides a context for assessing whether Kane's experience of detaching herself from her feelings and her fetus, but failing to prevent bonding with her unborn child, was an odd personal one. It helps us judge whether such an experience is unlikely to happen, for example, to more carefully screened birth mothers involved in surrogate contracts, or will quite likely face uncoerced women able to be in touch with their feelings. It looks as if the negative effects on the mother ought not to be discounted. Nor, given the growing knowledge of the incredibly complex development of the fetus, ought the negative impacts on the newborn to be forgotten. Thus, the argument from feelings, when explored, does not support surrogacy, but rather turns up pain and risks for the birth mother and infant, as well as the manipulation of frustrated longings by the baby brokers who promote and profit from it.

Rights

Another line of argument that some find persuasive stresses rights. Some proponents base the case for supporting surrogate motherhood on the liberal claim of respect for the rights and freedom of the individual as the supreme aim of a civilized society. Their view assumes, first, that the individual has the right to create a child as a form of self-expression and fulfilment and, if lacking procreative capacity or opportunity, has a claim on medical assistance and a third party with whom he or she has no relationship; and secondly, that adults enjoy the right and freedom to make contracts concerning the use of their procreative powers by persons enjoying no permanent relationship with them. These assumptions posit that others — society and the state? — have obligations, and that the creation of children can, for the sake of adults' wishes, beneficially be extracted from marriage and family. The child is assumed to be the means to the adults' ends. All of these assumptions seem dubious from either a human rights or a Christian perspective.

The rights of any individual must stop where the rights of others begin. Otherwise there is no protection for human dignity or life itself. And children — even newborns — ought to be accorded full human rights, as persons beginning the human adventure. Of course the idea that children have rights marks an important and very recent step forward in the world's history. But, in all the sympathizing with childless couples, who thinks of the rights of children, which are in issue and which are being violated in surrogate motherhood? The proposition that a woman may create a child to give to another for monetary return implies that she has ownership of that child. Parents do not own children. Children exist in their own right, they are a gift and a trust. In our common law legal tradition, parents enjoy rights in respect of their infant progeny so as to fulfil responsibilities to them, and children cannot be treated as chattels. It seems regressive in the extreme to propose that they now in surrogacy become their mother's possession and objects for their father's purchase. To propose that legal protection be afforded to adults acting on this tyrannical assumption of ownership is to take a giant step away from children's rights.

Nor can it be argued, as proponents of surrogacy assert, that the payment is for a service provided by the woman, not for the baby. As the Baby M case showed, under the contract she receives no compensation if she miscarries before the fifth month of pregnancy, only $1,000 if there is a miscarriage or stillbirth thereafter, and full payment only when the baby acknowledged by its father is transferred to him. "There is *no* reasonable doubt that what is being paid for is a child, *not* an egg, gestation, and childbirth 'services'." Nor can one legitimately argue in surrogacy that a father cannot purchase his own biological, genetically related child since it is already his, for, manifestly, "the child would not have existed at all but for the promise" of payment.[65]

Why should it be thought socially beneficial to encourage a woman to plan to set aside the commitment to the dependent infant of her body that is still society's best guarantee for its care? In surrogate motherhood her decision to conceive is one with the intention to divest herself of care of the infant she so creates. Why is society better for enabling women to conceive children as a money-making venture and bargain away the commitment to their care that has a visceral basis in bonding? Why is surrogate motherhood portrayed as liberal and humane? In the name of creating a baby, even if usually for a childless couple, it in fact reinforces men's rights. In effect it enables men, through contracts and the provision of sperm, to reclaim the rights to the custody of children which women, who bear all the labour of procreation, have only in this past century begun to share.

The whole idea of surrogate motherhood depends on a cerebral understanding of human nature that does not fit reality. The surrogate is required to regard the new life within her as the child of others, not herself. But this denial, enshrined in the abstractions of the commercial contract, flies in the face of women's experience of closeness in pregnancy, the true one-flesh unity. Mrs. Whitehead has agonizingly shown us that such a contract is a Faustian bargain — a sale of her soul. In making her rational agreement, she bargained that her will and mind could rule the feelings that come with one of the most intense creative experiences a woman can have. But since woman — like man — is a thinking being, not schizoid body/mind, the bargain proved folly. Such a contract could make sense only if human nature were dualistic, if the mind ran the body as the driver the car. The assumption that human beings are wholly rational and governed by their will is a key one in the Cartesian philosophy that undergirds our society, but human experience shows it to be false. We are whole persons and deny the mystery of our emotions and souls to our peril. The equally false but prevalent Cartesian assumption that reason, technology, and rational mechanisms bring progress is in the instance of surrogacy also disproved.

Thus the rights argument misunderstands human nature and degrades it. Through it women, children, and in the end, men are exploited and demeaned.

Honouring Our Humanness

What is the way forward through the maze of claimed rights and conflicting feelings, the way that will make and keep life human, that will honour and support our humanness? Anglicans apply the tests of reason, tradition, and scripture. We have a holistic understanding of human nature — woman and man are embodied selves. Whether we begin with reflection on the virgin mother and the Christ child, common sense, or science, isn't the bond born of pregnancy, and the strong impulse to nurture that accompanies it, an intrinsic part of human life to be valued? Isn't the commitment of a mother to her child a mark of our humanness? Such a natural bond and commitment may break down or have to be set aside. But to posit as moral, socially good, and worthy of legal protection, an approach to parenthood that requires a woman to consent to abandon the life created in the same moment that she chooses to create it is to poison the wellsprings of our humanity.

The Faustian bargain that reason dictate emotion and control her attachment to her own flesh *can* be carried out — human nature is plastic. Social coercion and approval can bring women's needs to converge on surrogacy as the fulfilment of femininity and the resolution of conflict by their own consent to be infantilized as "surrogate" mothers. But the dualism inherent in rational contracting about the intimate experience of childbearing, which enmeshes body, mind, and spirit, is not consonant with human nature if that nature is as Christians understand it. The very notion of making an informed, irrevocable contract — a notion dear to legal advocates of surrogate motherhood — is folly where complex and ambivalent feelings are involved. Reason cannot be king in realms of deepest human intimacy. Unless it be with incalculable and entirely avoidable pain and grief, in the betrayal of our humanity.

The church which long reinforced male domination, in the past taught female submission, defined woman by her biology, diminished her horizons, and promoted pro-natalism must recognize that justice requires us to reject the stereotypical thinking about women and their fulfilment which lies behind surrogate motherhood. Since women, everywhere, are treated as second-class citizens, in its commitment to social justice the church must name the social coercion and economic exploitation inherent in surrogacy. It is time to call a halt to asking women to live out self-giving by double duty in creating children for others. In a society in which men earn 50 per cent more than women, and women, with inadequate social assistance, often have a tough time providing for their children, women can be forced to accept that doing their all for their family necessitates becoming a surrogate mother for someone wealthier. Her body, mind, and soul, her personhood can be made a bargaining tool in tough times. So it is necessary to stand up for the humanity, dignity, and wholeness of women. And we must think of the children, who are pawns in this new adults' roulette: they need protection.

The biblical call is to justice and love. Justice requires us to treat every person as a bearer of dignity, of the image of God. Love can be fulfilled only if we do unto others as we would have them do unto us. But love cannot be hired, it can only be given and received.

If we are to remain in the ethical tradition of the Anglican Church of Canada, affirmed in our studies on abortion and sexuality, we must approach the ethical issues taking into account the widest net of facts, feelings, and rights. Testing these realities by scriptural values and theological insights, we should identify surrogate motherhood as corrosive of our very humanness. It is not of the things that make and keep us human.

Notes

1. "Grandmom, triplets 'fine' after extraordinary surrogate birth," *Toronto Star*, 2 Oct. 1987.
2. Stephen Wilson, "Surrogate birth riles public," *Ottawa Citizen*, 5 Nov. 1988.
3. "Surrogate motherhood: is it a good idea?" *Chatelaine*, September 1987, p. 38.
4. Darcy Henton, "Pickering couple Canada's 1st to get surrogate to bear embryo," *Toronto Star*, 14 May 1988. Bernard M. Dickens, a Toronto law professor, also says private arrangements between relatives and friends are being made. *See* Nomi Morris, "Province reviewing policies on surrogate motherhood," *Toronto Star*, 4 Oct. 1987.
5. Brian Goldman, "Infertility giving birth to new problems for doctors and lawyers," *Canadian Medical Association Journal*, vol. 138 (15 Jan. 1988), p. 167. Epstein himself has termed surrogacy "a morally bankrupt idea." *See* Dorothy Lipovenko, "Whose baby is it?" *Globe and Mail* (Toronto), 24 Jan. 1987.
6. Margrit Eichler and Phebe Poole, *The incidence of preconception contracts for the production of children among Canadians: a report prepared for the Law Reform Commission of Canada* (Toronto: Ontario Institute for Studies in Education, September 1988).
7. Quoted in Dorothy Lipovenko, "Study undertaken for law reform body turns up 118 surrogate-mother cases," *Globe and Mail*, 10 Feb. 1989, A1, A2.
8. Noel P. Keane with Dennis L. Breo, *The surrogate mother* (New York: Everest House, 1981), especially pp. 20-30, 224, 258, 265, 311, 313.
9. "Surrogate motherhood: is it a good idea?" *Chatelaine*, September 1987, pp. 38-39.
10. "Surrogate mothers: not so novel after all," *Hastings Center Report*, October 1983, pp. 28-29, 33. As sociologist Christine Overall notes, in *Ethics and human reproduction: a feminist analysis* (Boston: Allen & Unwin, 1987), p. 115, if she becomes pregnant at the first attempt of artificial insemination, her pay is about $1.50 per hour for a 24-hour-per-day 9-month job.
11. K.M. Brophy, "A surrogate mother contract to bear a child," *Journal of Family Law*, vol. 20 (1981-82), pp. 263-78.
12. Lori Andrews, *New conceptions: a consumer's guide to the newest infertility treatments* (New York: Ballantine Books, 1984), pp. 3, 181, 190, 194, 202, 215.

13. Lori Andrews, *Between strangers: surrogate mothers, expectant fathers, & brave new babies* (New York: Harper & Row, Publishers, 1989), pp. xii, 66, 71-73, 85, 91-94, 160, 225, 253-55.
14. P.G. O'Brien, "Surrogate motherhood: Uncertain status," *Ladies Home Journal*, February 1989, p. 28. Andrews also thinks that allowing people to sell their body parts would be a progressive step — see her article "My body, my property," *Hastings Center Report*, October 1986, pp. 28-38.
15. Susan Ince calls her "the happy hooker with a heart of gold," in "Inside the surrogate industry," a brilliant investigative piece in *Test-tube women: what future for motherhood*, edited by Rita Arditti, R.D. Klein, and Shelley Minden (London: Pandora Press, 1984), p. 115.
16. Handel is quoted to this effect in Gena Corea, *The mother machine: Reproductive technologies from artificial insemination to artificial wombs* (New York: Harper & Row, 1985), pp. 216-18, and also Andrews, *Between strangers*, p. 82.
17. Iwan Davies, "Contracts to bear children," *Journal of Medical Ethics* (London), vol. 11 (1985), p. 61.
18. *In the matter of Baby M*, A-39-87, Feb. 3, 1988, pp. 4-5, 53-54, 79; note 11 at pp. 54-55 outlines legal judgments in surrogate motherhood cases in both the U.S. and the United Kingdom.
19. G.J. Annas, "The baby broker boom," *Hastings Center Report*, June 1986, pp. 30-31.
20. G.J. Annas, "Death without dignity for commercial surrogacy: the case of Baby M," *Hastings Center Report*, April/May 1988, pp. 22-23 for all quotes in the para. thus far.
21. G.J. Annas, "Baby M: babies (and justice) for sale," *Hastings Center Report*, June 1987, p. 15.
22. Sherman Elias and G.J. Annas, "Social policy considerations in non-coital reproduction," *Journal of the American Medical Association*, vol. 255 no. 1 (3 Jan. 1986), p. 67.
23. Daniel Callahan, "Surrogate motherhood: a bad idea," *New York Times*, 20 Jan. 1987.
24. H.T. Krimmel, "The case against surrogate parenting," *Hastings Center Report*, October 1983, p. 36.
25. "Ethical considerations of the new reproductive technologies," *Fertility and Sterility*, vol. 46 no. 3, *Supplement 1* (September 1986), pp. 62s-67s. The American College of Obstetricians and Gynecologists, the American Medical Association, and the British Royal College of

Obstetricians and Gynaecologists have all expressed negative views about surrogacy. *See* the New York State Task Force on Life and the Law's report, *Surrogate parenting: analysis and recommendations for public policy* (New York, May 1988), pp. 103-4.
26. "Revised new guidelines for the use of semen-donor insemination," *Fertility and Sterility*, vol. 49 no. 2 (February 1988), p. 211.
27. Dorothy Lipovenko, "Freeze donor sperm 6 months because of AIDS risk, MDs urged," *Globe and Mail*, 20 Oct. 1988, A5.
28. W.R. Frederick, R. Delapenha, G. Gray, W.L. Greaves, C. Saxinger, "HIV testing of surrogate mothers," *New England Journal of Medicine*, vol. 317 no. 21 (19 Nov. 1987), pp. 1351-52.
29. Dorothy Lipovenko, "Whose baby is it?" *Globe and Mail*, 24 Jan. 1987.
30. OLRC, *Report on human artificial reproduction and related matters* (Toronto: Ministry of the Attorney General, 1985), 2 vols., pp. 219, 281-85. The commission's vice-chairman, H. Allan Leal, a former member of the Primate's Task Force on Human Life, registered a dissenting opinion in the report. Negative views on surrogacy were expressed by the British Warnock Committee in its 1984 report, and in the 1982-84 reports of the Waller Committee in Victoria, Australia, the result being legislation prohibiting commercial surrogacy and declaring surrogate contracts unenforceable in both places. For a survey of reports worldwide, *see* LeRoy Walters, "Ethics and new reproductive technologies: an international review of committee statements," *Hastings Center Report*, June 1987, pp. 3-9; for a summary of the Warnock and Waller reports, *see Surrogate parenting*, pp. 97-98; for discussion of various reports, *see* OLRC *Report*, p. 295 ff.
31. *Les enjeux éthiques et juridiques des nouvelles technologies de reproduction: le rapport du comité du barreau du Québec*, avril 1988.
32. Michigan, Keane's home state, in June 1988 made for-profit surrogacy contracts a felony subject to five years in jail and a $50,000 fine. *See* "Michigan bans surrogate contracts yesterday," *Globe and Mail*, 28 June 1988. But, according to Lori Andrews, on 19 Sept. 1988 a Michigan county circuit court judge approved an interpretation of that law which "allowed payment to surrogate mothers but gave her time after the baby's birth to change her mind and seek custody," and this interpretation, proposed by the attorney general and the American Civil Liberties Union (which had filed suit to declare the statute unconstitutional), makes commercial surrogacy legal in Michigan. *See Between strangers*, p. 271.

36 Whose Child Is This?

33. *Surrogate parenting*, pp. 25, 99, 116-20, 125.
34. *The mother machine*, material from Corea being drawn especially from pp. 7, 214, 216, 222-23, 227-28, 234, 288.
35. Overall, *Ethics and human reproduction*, p. 127 points out that when women are paid for their reproductive services, they are defined and used as a sex class and "the individual woman becomes a fiction."
36. Jeremy Rifkin of the Foundation on Economic Trends, whose members include leading American feminists, told the U.S. subcommittee on transportation, tourism and hazardous materials on 15 Oct. 1987: "If this new industry is permitted to grow, within a decade, thousands of poor women in this country and around the world will be used as 'breeding stock' to gestate babies for those who can afford the service. . . . Childbirth will become a lucrative new biotechnology industry." For this statement, *see* Eichler and Poole, *Incidence of preconception contracts*, appendix.
37. Susan Crean, in her book *In the name of the fathers: the story behind child custody* (Toronto: Amanita, 1988), pp. 19-22, says that in Canada the slow process of women's acquiring slivers of rights to their offspring began in Upper Canada in 1858. But not until 1917 was there a statute recognizing that parents have an equal right to custody of their children. This statute was in British Columbia, Ontario's came six years later, New Brunswick's several decades after that.
38. Ann Rauhala, "Hazards of surrogacy cited in report," *Globe and Mail*, 31 Aug. 1988, A9.
39. "Surrogate motherhood: is it a good idea?" *Chatelaine*, September 1987, pp. 38-39.
40. Sidney Callahan, "Lovemaking & babymaking, ethics & the new reproductive technology," *Commonweal*, 24 April 1987, pp. 236, 238.
41. Katha Pollitt, "Contracts and apple pie: the strange case of Baby M," *The Nation*, 23 May 1987, pp. cover, 684, 686.
42. Phyllis Chesler, *Sacred bond: the legacy of Baby M* (New York: Times Books, 1988), pp. 13, 16, 22, 44, 46, 60.
43. Congregation for the Doctrine of the Faith, "Instruction on respect for human life in its origin and on the dignity of procreation: replies to certain questions of the day," *Crux*, March 30, 1987, pp. 4-5, 14, 16.
44. "Report on health," *Blue book*, pp. 133, 141, Resolution #A-66.
45. *Blue book*, pp. 141-42, Resolution #A-89.
46. *Personal origins* (London: Working party on human fertilisation and embryology of the Board for Social Responsibility, 1985), pp. 41, 47.

47. "Synod's support for controlled embryo research," *Church Times* (London), 19 Feb. 1988.
48. *Making babies: the test tube and Christian ethics*, edited by Alan Nichols and Trevor Hogan (Canberra: Acorn Press, 1984), p. 3.
49. Andrews, *New Conceptions*, p. 86.
50. Annas, "Death . . . for commercial surrogacy," *Hastings Center Report*, April/May 1988, p. 22.
51. Andrews, *Between strangers*, p. 218.
52. *See*, for example, Louise Richards, "Giving the gift of life," *Ladies Home Journal*, February 1989, pp. 22, 28.
53. Sidney Katz, "The new reproductive era: Doctors will face ethical challenges," *Canadian Medical Association Journal*, vol. 136 (15 June 1987), p. 1293.
54. Elizabeth Kane, *Birth mother: the story of America's first legal surrogate mother* (New York: Harcourt Brace Jovanovich Publishers, 1988), pp. 27, 178. A recent study using questionnaires to 154 women and 64 men has confirmed earlier 1980s findings that the imaging of the fetus in ultrasound examinations, now common in pregnancy, enhances maternal bonding and attachment, by concretizing the baby. *See* Claude Villeneuve, C. Laroche, A. Lippman, and M. Marrache, "Psychological aspects of ultrasound imaging during pregnancy," *Canadian Journal of Psychiatry*, vol. 33 (August 1988), pp. 530-35.
55. Elizabeth Kane, "Elizabeth Kane and Mary Beth Whitehead: sisters in pain," *Redbook*, April 1988, pp. 144, 158.
56. *Birth mother*, pp. 275, 286, 289. Mary Beth Whitehead-Gould's own book, *A mother's story*, was published in 1989 by St. Martin's Press, New York.
57. OLRC *Report*, p. 231.
58. "Maternal attachment to the unborn child: a comparative study," pp. 42, 165, 179. Other studies the thesis cites include D.G. Benfield et al. 1976, J.H. Kennell et al. 1970, and J. Lumley 1980.
59. *Parenting your unborn child: a practical guide and permanent keepsake* (Toronto: Doubleday Canada Limited, 1988). p. 33.
60. A.J. DeCasper and W.P. Fifer, "Of human bonding: newborns prefer their mothers' voices," *Science*, vol. 208 (6 June 1980), pp. 1174-76.
61. *See The secret life of the unborn child* (New York: Delta, 1981), especially pp. 22-23, where Verny tells the story of Canadian conductor Boris Brott, who claims that "music has been a part of me since before birth." Brott says that as a young man he learned that pieces he could

play sight unseen had been ones his cellist mother had practised during her pregnancy.
62. *See* especially pp. 15, 24, 27, 81, 201.
63. *See Abortion, an ethical discussion* (London: Church Assembly Board for Social Responsibility, 1965), p. 37; Daniel Callahan, *Abortion: law, choice and morality* (London: Macmillan, 1970), pp. 57-58, citing studies.
64. Hilary Mackenzie, "Canada's first is due any day: 'rent-a-womb' birth kicks up controversy," *Globe*, 17 June 1982, pp. 1-2.
65. Annas, "Baby M," *Hastings Center Report*, June 1987, p. 14.

Reflections on the Significance and Meaning of Surrogate Motherhood*

Marsha Hewitt

Social analysis, if it hopes to be adequate to its task, must be able to name, or define as accurately as possible, the phenomenon it seeks to understand. This involves challenging the common, accepted explanation of social and cultural reality in order to see through to its actuality. Human beings cannot possibly understand the world they produce or find their bearings in it unless they are able to *name* it. The capacity to name a thing allows for critique, which helps to expose that which is problematic in society and detrimental to human well-being, so that alternatives may be posed. The capacity to name indicates the capacity to conceptualize — to think about the meaning of human experience and action. One of the peculiar contradictions facing human beings in this historical period is the disjunction between their technical abilities and their capacity for knowing how to think about, or make sense of, those abilities. We need a clear sense of the meaning of those technological developments which occur and continue to occur with such astonishing speed.

Human technical achievements, particularly in such areas as bio-medical and reproductive technology, threaten to make humanity into a stranger to itself, because what is ultimately at stake is not only the kind of world we wish to live in, but our very human self-image. Bio-medical and reproductive technology presents human beings with seemingly infinite possibilities

---

* A revised version of this essay appears in the Spring 1990 issue of the *Toronto Journal of Theology* under the title, ''Where Speech Has Lost Its Power'': A Social Ethical Reflection on the Meaning of Surrogate Motherhood.

to extend and create life, yet it leaves the question of the quality of human life unanswered. This question directly opens another, which is the *meaning* of human life, and human relationships.

The sophisticated achievements in reproductive technology, the apparent goal of which is to solve the painful problem of human "infertility," challenge our concepts and experience of our most intimate human relationships, in particular the relationships between men and women, and parents and their children. For example, *in vitro* fertilization, while offering one possible solution to infertility, poses a potential crisis within human relations and human self-understanding: by the technical means of *in vitro* fertilization, a woman may give birth to her own grandchildren, so that her daughter's children would also be her daughter's siblings.[1] What sense are people to make of themselves in such a situation? If human beings are indeed social beings who come to know themselves in and through their relations with others, then self-identity is deeply embedded in that complex of interrelationships. When that nexus of relationships is profoundly rearranged, people may experience overwhelming, irresoluble confusion concerning their very self-understanding.

Reproductive medical techniques, such as artificial insemination by donor, embryo transfer, egg donation, *in vitro* fertilization, and even so-called surrogate motherhood challenge and possibly undermine normative concepts of human self-identity. Since the relationship between parent and child is primary, we must consider what is constitutive of parenthood. The fact of being a parent brings with it the responsibility to know what is the meaning of parenthood, which is one of the most significant mediations of self-understanding. The various methods devised by medical science to solve the problem of infertility may leave human beings deeply mystified as to who, in the final analysis, they really are, because of the deeper confusion surrounding the question of to whom they belong. Mystification of this sort is bound to produce self-alienation.

One example of such mystification can be found in the language used to describe the phenomenon of surrogate motherhood. The woman who bears a child (for a fee) for another person or couple is commonly — but wrongly — called the "surrogate" mother. According to the *OED*, a surrogate is "a person appointed by authority to act in the place of another; a person or (usually) a thing that acts for or takes the place of another; a substitute, taking the place of or standing in for something else; representative; (v.) to appoint as a successor, substitute or deputy; to substitute in respect of a right or claim.'' A woman who gives birth to a child can hardly be a surrogate; indisputably, she *is* the mother, whether she decides to keep her child with her or not.

A surrogate normally pertains to a *function* or *thing* that replaces another function or thing, designated by some external authority. When applied to a pregnant woman, the definition of surrogacy means that a human being and her child are reduced to the twofold instrumentality of function and thinghood. The logic of surrogacy goes like this: the woman is appointed by a man to function reproductively for another woman who cannot (or will not) become pregnant herself, in order to produce a baby that will be *his* biological offspring. What results is a double thingification of both woman and child: a woman is hired for her reproductive labour power, to produce a suitable commodity — a human child — for sale/consumption. The woman turns herself into a self-contained assembly line through the hiring out of her uterus which grows and incubates a child that will fetch a price *if* it conforms to certain standards of quality production. The woman who hires herself out in this manner then is most accurately known in accordance with her function; a paid, contracted baby-producer. The man provides a part of the means of production with his sperm, and she provides the remainder not only with her reproductive organs, but her entire body — *soma* and *psyche*. She contributes the blood supply, the oxygen, the hormones — the technical means of production necessary to making a child. The woman is a paid wage-labourer whose product will be appropriated by her employer upon completion. Like any wage-labourer, the woman re-productive worker has no control over the use her product is put to once it goes to the market and is consumed. Like any other wage-labourer, the woman is alienated from the object of her productive activity, but in her particular case, there is a further alienation because her product is literally, physically, part of her. The woman splits herself off from herself, objectifying her body into an instrument of technical reproduction along with her child, which becomes a commodity item. But she is not even a surrogate mother, because what kind of mother can she be if she agrees to be reduced to a mere technical means of child production? The surrogate mother is the woman who assumes the role of mother (in place of the birth mother) after the sperm-provider and employer has appropriated the product of the child-producer's labour. Both the birth mother and the surrogate function in relation to the child (in their various ways) through the man, whose initial rights of appropriation and role in relation to both women and the child are basically no different from those of any employer.

In order to explore the deeper meaning of surrogate motherhood, it is necessary to analyze its socio-economic mediations. The primary mediation of surrogate motherhood in advanced industrial capitalist society concerns the techniques and relations of commercial production. The relations among the people involved in commercial surrogate contracts parallel those of industrial production models. Baby production for market consumption and profit effects the rationalization of human relations according to industrial activity, so that the potential human qualities in those relationships are called into question. For efficiency's sake, the baby producer must not regard her product as her baby or child and indeed dare not since she is producing it for sale. Moreover, it is entirely contrary to the inherent logic or rationale of the situation to regard the child as hers; for her to do so involves quite a different order of rationality in which the mother understands herself as a living subject, and her child as an end in itself, not a means for profit. The surrogate contract arrangement is the negation of the full humanity and subjectivity of both the woman and child. The woman is objectified in and through her function and role of employee whose sole purpose is to fulfil the demands of her employer. Since contracts imply legal agreements, possible punishments or penalties may ensue if a contract is broken without mutual agreement between the parties. In other words, a woman is open to penalty if she realizes herself as the *mother* of her child in a commercial surrogate arrangement.

If a woman changes her mind and decides she does not want to sell the baby after all, then she upsets the entire arrangement by introducing a different rationality into the situation, and thus acts "irrationally" in the context of the contractual agreement. The logic of instrumentality belongs to a contrary order of rationality to that which is inherent in genuinely human relations. If the woman changes her mind, she attempts to humanize the relation between herself and her child, thus introducing a set of values which negate those upon which the contract is based. The relations between surrogate mother and the man who employs her presume the objectified nature of all concerned: the employer, who provides part of the means of baby production with his sperm and puts up the money for the final product so that he is more of a progenitor than a father; the woman, who contracts not only her womb, but whole body as the main part of the means of production, while implicitly attempting to deny her motherhood; and the baby, who is the most objectified of all, since s/he is the sale item, and totally involuntarily.

The surrogate mother phenomenon clearly demonstrates the pervasive power of the market mentality to penetrate the most intimate areas of human relations; we can only conclude that the deliberate production of babies as market commodities inescapably demonstrates the ruthless logic of a consumer-oriented society, which is that everything is for sale. Furthermore, when we recognize and acknowledge capitalism's inexhaustible drive to expand and create new markets, then the commodification of the human being is perfectly, but tragically, logical and inevitable. Human beings, as the objects of their own production, consume *themselves* in the market which becomes the main arena of human action.

A Biblical Precedent?

Could it not be argued that the bearing of children for others is an old practice in most societies, and that commercial surrogacy is just a modern version of what has gone on for a very long time? What, it may be asked, is so different and so unacceptable about present-day surrogate arrangements? One might point to the story of Ishmael as a case in point. However, a brief consideration of the main features of the biblical story of Hagar and Ishmael rather highlights the radical negativity of contemporary surrogate contracts. The main outline of the story is that Hagar is an Egyptian slave owned by Sarah, who cannot conceive. In order to ensure the continuation of her husband Abraham's line, Sarah offers that Hagar be his concubine. Hagar becomes pregnant and has a son, Ishmael. Later Sarah herself gives birth to a son, Isaac, and eventually expels Hagar and Ishmael from her household in order to ensure Isaac's inheritance as Abraham's legitimate heir. Even though Hagar is a slave from a foreign people, at no point is her motherhood of Ishmael in question. Sarah does not take Ishmael away from Hagar, nor does Abraham. Because she is a slave and then concubine of Abraham, Hagar is a legitimate member of his household, however inferior her status. Abraham is responsible for Hagar and Ishmael's well-being, and even when he agrees to turn them out, he gives them some provisions for their survival.

The point is that, however low Hagar's status is in Abraham's household, there remains some human element in the relations between Abraham, Hagar, and Ishmael. In the first instance, Ishmael is born as the result of a sexual relation between his mother and father, and not through medical techniques; Hagar and Ishmael are cared for by Abraham, and there is some indication in the biblical text that he looks kindly on both mother and son. Even Sarah, who becomes abusive of Hagar, at no point denies Hagar's relationship to Ishmael and no attempt is made to separate the boy from his mother. Whatever problems exist in this story, the relations between these people are recognizably human, and each has feelings for and about the others.

The development from the economy of slavery to wage labour under a capitalist market economy undermines the human element within social relations, with the result that cash and contracts become the central features and aim of human relations. It is precisely the element of cash, or wages, that threatens the human quality of social relations in order to produce the efficient impersonality that characterizes the employer/employee connection. But how would the story of Hagar read in contemporary times, and in the context of surrogate motherhood contracts? Certainly it would mean something quite different in our society, and in spite of the same formal relationships existing between the people, Abraham would have contracted with Hagar, probably through an agency, to become pregnant through artificial insemination. He would provide the sperm, she the rest of the necessary materials. Then Abraham would have bought Ishmael for a few thousand dollars, Sarah would have raised him, and Hagar would have conveniently disappeared. Rendered in this way, the story of Hagar is utterly transformed, although the plot structure remains the same. What transforms the story is the socio-economic mediation of the relations between the people, which is decisive for a clear understanding of it. In the biblical account, God came to the aid of Hagar and Ishmael as they were dying of thirst in the desert. Abraham is dear to God, and specifically chosen by God in a covenant relationship. One of the reasons why God helps them is because of the human bonds between the people; Ishmael is, after all, Abraham's first-born son, and Hagar is his mother. Thus she is intimately connected to Abraham, her banishment notwithstanding. In our time, there would be no need of God's intervention whatsoever, partly because no one goes thirsty with ten thousand dollars in the bank, and Ishmael would grow up with all the comforts of a middle-class household. Given that in our world the parties enter into a business contract which terminates upon delivery of the approved product, there is little that is human in this limited, artificial, and technical arrangement. With the disappearance of the distinctively human from social relations, what place is there for God within a cold cash nexus? Relations based upon a calculus of exchange exclude both the human and the divine.

The Commodification of Women's Bodies

The production of children for sale logically extends a particular condition of women that is historically long standing: the commodification of their bodies. Pornography provides a useful analogy for further probing the meaning of surrogate motherhood. The commodification of women is at the core of both pornography and prostitution, in which women put their bodies, or more precisely — *specific body parts* — up for sale as market objects. Pornography reduces women to an abstract bodily form, which is further dispersed into bodily fragments. Pornography is obsessed with depersonalized breasts and genitalia in a manner quite divorced from the bodily integrity of women. The woman's face is treated as little more than a plastic appendage, which usually bears a silly expression that conceals her specific personality. In pornography, woman is reduced to a standard physical type, which is also a degradation of both her body and her spirit. There is no possibility of considering woman as equally both body and spirit, a notion which is reinforced by traditional Christian anthropology. In such Christianity, women are most often associated with the corporeal, the animal, and thus demonic spheres. Their full human potential and meaning is treated as nearly identical with their biological capacities, so there is very little room to view women as intellectual, moral, and spiritual beings. In the prevailing Christian world view, female ontology is firmly rooted in corporeal, corrupted nature. Contemporary pornography is the visual representation of this view, yet in a totally secularized and mercantile way. The specifically religious beliefs underlying these negative attitudes to women may have long since been forgotten, but nonetheless this misogynistic residue remains within our larger culture. Thus, woman cannot be taken seriously as a human being, otherwise she could not be used as an effective mechanism for the acquisition of profit. Here too we see woman as thing, a means of production, the product of which is herself, split into pieces, reduced to incoherency, but generating huge profit for the pornography industry.

A similar case can be made in the case of prostitution, in which the woman rents a part of her physical self for another's use. Again, her human value is translated into cash, which is true of all commodity value. The relation between the prostitute and her client is one of instrumental, impersonal genital and monetary exchange. Prostitution is wage labour in one of its more degrading forms, and has little if anything to do with sex, at least for the woman.

Viewed within the overall framework of the sex industry, we can see the phenomenon of turning one's womb into a machine for baby production is simply another form of the commodification of women that already exists in pornography and prostitution. The only difference between women employed in pornography and prostitution and those who bear and sell children for others is that they work in different branches of what is essentially the same industry, with its specific forms of division of labour. The reproduction industry may be reasonably understood as a sub-industry of the larger sex-industry. What all these women have in common is that the nature of the work they do involves a degree of literal self-commodification that reduces their human essence to mere bodily functions. To do this work effectively and efficiently involves the development of a particular kind of self-consciousness that participates in the instrumentalization of the woman herself and the object of her production.

She must objectify herself in the way she is already objectified if she is to do her job.

For example, one surrogate mother stated that she had to "condition" herself not to become attached to the child she was carrying for another.[2] This was a lower working-class woman who needed the money to help support her family because her husband's wages were insufficient. Part of her self-conditioning involved her understanding her work as presenting a childless couple with the "gift" she had made them. However, a gift is something freely given, for which the receiver pays nothing. But even as gift the child she had was still an object, and the fact that the woman received payment for the child exposes the discourse of gift-giving as simply empty self-deception.

When women contract themselves out for reproductive labour, they open themselves to the same kind of exploitation usually associated with wage-labour relations. If a woman receives $10,000 (the most common price to date) for her work, she is earning about $1.50 an hour, 24 hours per day. Others who profit from her work (the middle-man) earn far more than she does. Not only does she produce a baby for sale, but in so doing, she also generates profit for the baby-broker who arranges the whole surrogacy arrangement. In order to ensure a high quality product for the buyer, the woman may become vulnerable to many specific forms of possible domination, i.e., must she follow rules about eating, drinking, smoking, sleeping, exercise, etc.? What rights does the buyer potentially have over her daily living behaviour? And if the product is defective, the woman may easily find herself in the position of caring for a retarded or deformed person for the rest of her life. Since most surrogate mothers belong to lower working-class households, such an event could be an overwhelming burden for her and her family. Seen from this perspective, surrogate motherhood represents a further exploitation of working-class and poor women, not to mention the potential labour force of poverty-stricken women in the world, who would certainly be paid much less in a surrogacy arrangement than a North American.

An analysis of contract maternity within the context of industrial, capitalist, consumerist society shows it to be a deepening of the objectivation, commodification, and material exploitation of women. The woman as baby-producer is little more than an object of use-purchase by men; this amounts to reproductive prostitution. Prostitutes are among the most despised, most often penalized and preyed upon people in society. Because of the nature of their work, they are interchangeable and of course disposable; any female can do it. They are tools of another's use, as are surrogates, who are tools of reproductive use for someone else. In the same fashion as prostitutes, surrogate mothers are also interchangeable and disposable, precisely because their value is defined within the female's reproductive bodily function. As long as she has a normally functioning reproductive system, any woman is a possible candidate for the position of surrogate mother. Should she in some way fail her function, she will be discarded and replaced by another mechanism which hopefully will not malfunction.

Women's "Liberation" in the Context of Biological Determinism

It is highly significant that a society which in many ways acknowledges women's rights, however painstakingly and reluctantly, doggedly refuses to permit women's bodily self-determination. The abortion controversy provides another helpful analogy which further illustrates this curious contradiction. It is often argued that the issue at the centre of the abortion battle is deeper than women's rights to abortion, but is rather the right to consciously direct one's life.[3] Margaret Sanger, a women's rights activist of the turn of the century, stated the issue like this: "No woman can call herself free who does not own or control her body. No woman can call herself free until she can choose consciously whether she will or will not be a mother."[4] There are many women who share Sanger's view. However, the point made by Sanger goes beyond the issue of abortion to raise the question of what motherhood means to a woman, and under what circumstances becoming a mother enhances the humanity of the woman, her family, and the community. Do women have children as the result of a free, loving decision, or because, for instance, they need money, which is an indirect form of coercion. Economic necessity can be another way by which a woman feels forced to have a child if the society allows her to sell the child through a commercial surrogate agreement. Women's not having access to abortion is another way whereby women may feel forced into having children they may not want. Despite the acceptability or unacceptability of abortion as such, the abortion controversy reveals deeper concerns, along with surrogate motherhood, showing how woman's reproductive capacity may be seen to be used against her.

Both questions about abortion and surrogate motherhood confront us with a more important question: under what circumstances and for what reasons ought new life to be brought into the world? The question as to the motivation to have a child has still not received the full attention it requires, and thus the more fundamental question of the meaning of parent-child relationships is pervaded by confusion. The Baby M case, in which the mother initially lost her parental rights, is a concrete example of possible conflicting motives and values around parenthood. By the time the case went to court, it appeared to be a contest between the male desire *to procreate* as against the woman's desire *to nurture*.[5] The affirmation of the desire of the male to reproduce (and thus claim custody on the basis of genetic links) is the direct negation of the already existing relationship and bond between the woman and her child, which is more than genetic. The right of the male to procreate was upheld in the Baby M case by the lower court, although another court decision granted the birth mother visiting rights. Nonetheless, the father won custody on the basis of his biological connection with the child. The final outcome of the Baby M case asks us to expand our concept of reproductive freedom to include both the actual giving birth to a child as well as the woman's right to raise and nurture that child. Surrogacy arrangements encourage the former, but seek to absolutely deny the latter. Thus the question of reproductive freedom for women includes the whole issue of surrogacy contracts. Commercial surrogate mother arrangements undermine women's capacity for free, autonomous personhood in relation to the bearing and nurturing of children. Furthermore, clarity around the motivation to create children is essential to the kind of value we place on children, as individuals and as a society. If the desire to have children is instrumentalized in any way, the child is in danger of being instrumentalized him or herself.

The practice of surrogate motherhood then has implications that go beyond issues concerning the condition of women. Surrogate motherhood is indicative of the deepening rationalization of society and humanity as such by extending the relations produced by the division of labour along industrial and technological lines, applied to the most intimate area of human relationships. Women who enter into maternity contracts for producing children for sale are subject to a 'de-skilling" of labour, as it were, similar to that which has been taking place in industry since the introduction of mass production techniques. For example, prior to the introduction of the assembly line, industrial workers were much more highly skilled, which meant they could exercise a higher degree of control over the production process than was possible with assembly-line production. With the introduction of the assembly line, the division of labour was elaborated into smaller and simpler tasks, resulting in a semi-skilled, cheap labour force that was dispensable and replaceable. Worker apprenticeship dwindled because a large number of highly skilled jobs were abolished. Furthermore, the de-skilling of labour allowed for far greater managerial control over the industrial workforce, because human labour became increasingly devalued as an activity involving the expertise and knowledge of the worker. In analogous fashion, something quite similar happens to women who contract themselves as surrogate mothers. The whole complex experience of becoming pregnant is hypostasized into a technical, commercial venture, whereby the woman merely offers her egg, uterus, and entire body to the reproduction process of a commodity item. The complex and intense nature of maternity, which includes long-term responsibilities and an emotional, psychological relationship between the woman and her child, is abolished in the surrogate arrangement unless the woman changes her mind, as the birth mother did in the Baby M case.

The elaboration of the division of labour into more simplified, mindless tasks, along with the abolishment of labour altogether in many technological industries, has produced a social crisis that is showing few signs of improvement. People are becoming more atomized and alienated from each other, more instrumentalized, used and using each other as mere means. A woman who contracts to produce a baby for sale experiences all of this, but *within* herself. She must further instrumentalize herself (as she had already been instrumentalized from without), transforming her body into an object and means of production, generating profit for someone else. This process results in a profound alienation of herself from herself, which she must force herself to sustain, if the surrogacy agreement is to be protected.

Commercial Fatherhood

So far, this discussion has focused primarily on the woman who contracts to produce a baby in the surrogate arrangement. However, there is another important issue to be explored in order to fully comprehend the meaning of surrogate motherhood, and that is the nature of the relationships between the people involved. What are the common elements that mediate and thus bind the people together in commercial surrogate contracts? This question is important because the mediations define their relationships, and in particular, with the child, who is after all, the *object* of the whole enterprise. Finally, what is the key element that makes the surrogate arrangement even possible?

The most common type of surrogacy arrangement is initiated by a man who wants to procreate but for some reason is unable to do so with his wife. The surrogate arrangement allows him to fulfil his procreative desire by means of money. Without money, such a man would be unable to realize himself as a father. "Money is the *procurer* between man's need and the object," wrote Karl Marx, the nineteenth-century social philosopher, and that is precisely true in the surrogate mother contract agreement. Money nullifies the barrier between himself and the object he desires, which is his biological child. It is money that not only transforms him into a genetic father, but is also the original or generative bond between himself and his child, for the child is the object for which he made cash payment. The child is not the issue of the mutual love between the man and his wife, it is not the result even of sexual passion. Rather the child is the object of a business transaction between a buyer and seller. By means of money, the man achieves what is impossible on the human level — fatherhood, an added dimension to his self-identity.

Conversely, the same medium through which the man finds affirmation as father is that which negates the motherhood of the woman who bears his child. By the technical means of money, the woman may not (indeed, must not) regard herself as a mother or her child as *her* child. "*Money* as the external, universal *medium* and *faculty*, allows the man to turn his self-image as potential father into a reality, while transforming the reality of the woman's maternal relation to the child into a *mere image*."[6] Thus the woman is called surrogate so that her human connection with the child may be denied. She must relate to the child in terms of the mechanistic function of a thing. Thus the power that money effects through the "transformation of all human and natural properties into their contraries"[7] turns everything on its head, producing distortion and confusion in human relations precisely because, as the primary mediation of those relations in a market economy, money obliterates that which is human in social relations. Thus money as such represents the "alienated ability of mankind"[8] because it can do what an individual by his or her human powers alone cannot do: thus a person can become a biological parent for a price, and that same price can deny the parenthood of another person. Money, as the mediation and thus negation of genuinely human relationships, alters and undermines self-identity, the very self-image of being human. In commercial surrogacy contracts, children are not the result of love and passion between two people who wish to embody their relationship in a child; the child is the result of a business transaction, through which a man thinks he may become a father as long as the woman pretends that she is not the mother of the child she sells to him. In such arrangements, cash exchange actually produces what can only be called a grotesque lie. "Since money, as the existing and active concept of value, confounds and confuses all things, it is the general *confounding* and *confusing* of all things — the world upside-down — the confounding and confusing of all natural and human qualities."[9] The implications of surrogate motherhood, a contract by which a baby is made and then sold, penetrate far beyond the issue itself, exposing something fundamental about the nature and destiny of humanity in this historical period.

Conclusion

The point of this paper is to ask the question of the meaning of surrogate motherhood, and what this social phenomenon reveals to us about who we are and what we are becoming as human

— or inhuman — beings. One thing is clear: in the context of our contemporary market economy, surrogate contracts show us that everything has a price, including children. There was a time when the buying and selling of human beings was commonly known as slavery, and many societies viewed its abolition as a positive achievement.

In ethical terms, what language most accurately describes surrogate motherhood arrangements? As stated at the beginning of this paper, the question of language and naming is critical to the whole discussion of surrogacy. We must first know *what* we are dealing with before we can figure out *how* to deal with it.

Those who champion surrogate parenting see it as a service to people who need it. The largest surrogate parenting agency, The Infertility Centre of New York, advertises itself as offering "a practical alternative" to childless couples, and its founder refers to his "love and feelings"[10] for his own children as the reason for his founding the surrogate program. The brochure does not indicate how much money he makes for the privilege of being part of "the miracle" of providing people with children.

The primary motive of the commercial surrogate venture is profit, as is the case with any other business. The emotional pain that many people experience at not being able to have children has been transformed into a market with huge profit-making potential. Such a "solution" to "infertility" actually prevents people from overcoming their suffering, at not being able to have their own children, by offering an illusory solution — to those who can afford it. Surrogacy arrangements help no one to come to terms with their infertility, and so foreclose the possibility of seeing one's life and one's self in a healthier way. Surrogate contracts thus function to sustain the unacceptability of not being able to have children that many people experience. Not only are babies sold and bought in commercialized surrogacy; so is human pain, fear, guilt, and frustration. People who view their relationship as inadequate or somehow a failure by the absence of children unwittingly provide the entrepreneurs of surrogate-parenting operations with a monetary hunting-ground, whereby their pain is exploited for another's gain. The solution to infertility is not to be found then in surrogate mother transactions, but rather in human attitudes and self-understanding. The Christian churches, society, and individuals must re-think and re-evaluate their general attitude toward childlessness which interprets it as a failure or even curse. However disappointing it may be, the physical incapacity to bear children in no way indicates that a marriage or the individuals involved are in any way inadequate or intrinsically defective. As long as those kind of negative evaluations of the meaning of infertility go unchallenged, the buying and selling of children, along with the cynical exploitation of human pain, will continue and increase.

Notes

1. *Toronto Star*, 2 October 1987.
2. "A surrogate's story," *Time*, 10 September, p. 51.
3. Marsha Hewitt, "The remedy is desperate but sometimes, necessary," *Compass*, July 1988, pp. 32-34.
4. In Josephine Donovan, *Feminist Theory: The Intellectual Traditions of American Feminism* (New York: F. Ungar, 1986), p. 52.
5. Karl Marx and Friedrich Engels, *Collected Works* (New York: International Publishers, 1975), III, 1843-1844, p. 325.
6. Marx and Engels, p. 325.
7. Marx and Engels, p. 324.
8. Marx and Engels, p. 325.
9. Marx and Engels, p. 326.
10. Brochure of The Infertility Centre of New York.

"Rooted in Relation":
A Theological Reflection on Christian Values and Surrogacy

Don Thompson

A Method for Reflecting Theologically

When a society proposes a new social convention (in this case, surrogate motherhood) or use of a scientific or technological advance (such as ovum donation, embryo transfer, or sperm insemination), Christians in that society have to appraise it from the perspective of their faith tradition. The proposal may be entirely new, but the values it promotes should be consistent with those of the ongoing Christian tradition. For Anglicans, such values are initially drawn from scripture, but are continually understood afresh as the church lives and worships faithfully in each generation. The proposal of surrogacy, in which fertility techniques are to be used to enable an infertile couple to have a child genetically related to them but carried and birthed by another woman, we shall see represents a value structure quite foreign to this living faith tradition.

In the short sections that follow, we will explore several active Christian traditions that contain values which seem to challenge this new proposal of surrogacy. These will differ from chapter 4 of this report where Marsha Hewitt identifies the negative theological meaning which can be discerned in the proposal. In contrast, this chapter tries to identify some active theological traditions of the Christian heritage which would clearly challenge such a proposal by reaffirming the intentional unity of married relationship, sexual intimacy, and the procreation of children. Readers familiar with these traditions may wish to examine in detail only the concluding section of this chapter. It is there that the results of these several reflections are gathered together, giving an indication of the basic theological reasons why we should not support a proposal of surrogate motherhood within the Christian community represented by the Anglican Church of Canada.

Origins of the Covenant of Marriage: Genesis

Procreation and sexual partnership are foundationally linked through an understanding of the covenant of marriage, which is first of all proposed in Hebrew scripture and subsequently upheld in Christian scripture. The tribal and biblical convention of covenant describes a series of mutual pledges between two parties set in the context of a mutual story or act which highlights the meaning of the pledges. For Israel, the basic covenant comes through the event of safe delivery from oppression in Egypt, which was understood as a special blessing for Israel: "I shall be your God and you shall be my people" (Lev. 11:45, Jer. 7:21, Ezek. 36:28). The Ten Commandments in return became what Israel pledged to God. But there were other covenantal relationships and pledges as well, and one of the most central for us is the covenant of marriage. For the Judeo-Christian, this covenant links marriage, sexuality, and procreation in a specific relationship of mutuality. It is remarkably clear in its origin, as it has remained clear in its subsequent Jewish and Christian practice.

The covenant is embedded in the creation stories of Genesis. While our versions of them go back to the sixth century B.C. when Israel was in exile in Babylon, the stories themselves go back to the second millennium of early patriarchal history.

Most readers will have noticed that there are two separate creation stories: Genesis 1 ff. and Genesis 2.4 ff. These are different but not incompatible, and each is rich with meaning.[1]

In the first account, we witness the earth, seas, and skies created by the spirit (*ruah* in Hebrew, meaning *breath*) of God, out of a void or nothingness. Then beyond that physical world, the botanical and biological world are created (and related the first to the next), each being affirmed by God as "good." Related to that same order follows the creation of the human (*adham* in Hebrew, meaning human: without sexual distinction). In this account the human, being created "in the image of God," is created as both male and female (Gen. 1:28). The blessing of this covenant relationship is for the human to be created in the reflected image of God. As such, the human and the rest of creation are bound into an interrelatedness of "everything that has the breath of life" (Gen. 1:30), which itself is a mutual blessing for everything created. But man and woman are to make two pledges to God:

- to be fruitful,
- to have dominion (be custodian) over the fish of the sea, etc.

This is a covenant tradition of mutuality in which humans, understood as being in the image of God, are thereby entrusted with the responsibilities of procreation and care of the earth.

But in the second account of creation (Gen. 2:4), two further components are introduced into the covenantal relationship: sexuality and a partnership of marriage. Hardly has the physical creation been described before God introduces a specific quality to relatedness: sexual differentiation. But there is a very unique purpose indicated for this: "it is not good that the human (*adham*) should be alone; I will make for it a companion" (Gen. 2:18).

The word companion or helper (*ezer* in Hebrew) is one of mutuality and partnership, implying co-working and co-operation. But the creation needs another essential component: community. So that the human will not be alone, God develops further life — "every beast of the field and bird of the air" — for the help and companionship of the human. Yet amongst these, God finds no "fit" companion for intimacy with the human. To achieve this, God takes from the *adham* (which had been formed from dust and God's "breath of life") a bodily portion, and forms it into a companion portion. Only at this point in the Hebrew account does the word *adham* (human) shift to become the two interrelated words *ish* (man) and *ishish* (woman). Woman and man are created for each other. But the final line of the story is almost as important as all that has come before it, for in that one line are made clear all the social and cultural implications of marriage and family for future Jewish and Christian communities: "Therefore a man leaves his father and his mother and cleaves to his wife, and they become one flesh" (Gen. 2:24).

"One flesh" is a direct allusion to sexual intimacy. But in this story it is lifted up as the means of companionship, of not being alone, that God makes possible between two humans. This companionship of intimacy and sexuality is clear from the nakedness of the man and woman, and that they were "not ashamed" is a further indication that their sexuality is natural to God's intended companionship for them. Sexuality, then, is all part of the blessing of God's intended covenant for humankind. In return, the pledge required is "not to eat" of the tree of good and evil in the centre of the garden. Many generations have speculated on the meaning of this tree, but there seems to be agreement that it represents something capable of being given to humans (hence it is in the garden), yet it is reserved for giving only by God. What it seems to represent is that there are limits to what humans should do in the creation. As with the tree itself, the consequents are good and evil. But they do eat, and are subsequently banished from the garden: the man to the toil of work, the woman to the pain of birth. For both, sexuality as companionship turns out to have a negative side in isolation and a sense of shame. Yet the original intent of the blessing of the covenant remains with them: companionship and mutuality rather than isolation and shame.

Although biblical scholars have distinguished these two accounts, both Jewish and Christian traditions treat the accounts as one, and have identified in them a single covenantal relationship in which we understand that:

- humankind is blessed as a creation in the image of God,
- humankind is blessed with companionship, both in the biological world and, more significantly, in the sexual intimacy of woman and man,
- the companionship of humankind is blessed as the source of further human (pro)creation: children.

But as with every covenant, there are pledges or obligations:

- to be responsible for further procreation,
- to be custodian over the botanical and biological world,
- to be a companion with the biological world,
- not to do certain things reserved only for God,
- to be companion as woman and man,
- to leave original family, and become originating family.

There is a unity to this covenant in that it is uniformly relational. Humankind is related to God by being in the same image. Humankind is related to the creation itself. The biological world is companion to the human, and in relationship. With such relationship goes responsibility. But humankind is related to itself through sexual differentiation, to be a companion with itself through which it fulfills the mutual obligation of procreation.

Humankind thereby is part of a process, of the child nurtured by woman and man who are to be mother and father, subsequently to generate a new companionship of woman and man. In its initial form, the entire set of relationships is good, including the relationship of naked intimacy in which man and woman are not ashamed. This covenant from Genesis has remained normative for both Hebrew and Christian traditions over countless centuries; both traditions look to this account to clarify the meaning of being in covenant relationship.

What values, then, does this tradition have which might challenge the proposal of surrogate motherhood? These seem to be:

- human life is more than a mere entity of creation, having been created in the image of God;
- humankind is blessed with the relationship of woman and man in which companionship, sexuality, and procreation are blended in the unity of one flesh;
- humankind is not to do certain things reserved only for God (limitation);
- there are obligations to this covenant which pertain to a couple in relationship, their children, and the rest of created life.

The "New" Covenant: Related to Christ

In the account of Jesus whom we call the Christ, the original tradition of the Genesis covenant is clearly upheld. In the gospels of both Mark (10:8) and Matthew (19:5) the creation of male and female is recalled, but in the specific context that in relationship the two "become one body," and cannot become two again. Jesus was upholding the covenant of marriage which should not be abused. But the apostle Paul developed this still further, in recalling that "the two become one flesh" (I Cor. 6:17), with his notion of the church being related to Christ as bride and bridegroom. For Paul, marriage was the ultimate analogy for two entities achieving the unity of one, for the church and Christ become "one spirit" (I Cor. 6:17) in this union just as presumably women and men become "one flesh" in marriage. As it is put in the letter to the Ephesians: "This is a great mystery, and I take it to mean Christ and the church" (5:32). He assumes the mutuality of the marriage relationship itself in that both husband and wife are to live, nourish, and cherish each as their own flesh, because they are members now of the same body. In that sense, both are to "be subject to one another out of reverence for Christ" (5:21), the "other partner" of the couple in relationship. Paul has brought a new level of mutuality and respect to the tradition of the one flesh in Genesis, by the image of Christ and the church.

The apostle John adds still a further dimension to the relationship of one flesh located in the book of Genesis and reappropriated for Christians in Paul's writings. In John's narrative of creation, at the beginning of his gospel, he describes the presence of God as "the Word" (meaning Jesus) which has been present from the beginning. But, in an astounding assertion for the first-century hearers of this account, "The Word became flesh and dwelt among us" (Jn. 1:14). God has come in Jesus the Christ, and thereby continues to come to every woman and man as "the true light" that enlightens everyone (1:9). By the coming of Christ which we have come to call the Incarnation, we understand God to have entered affirmatively into all of human life and flesh. As such, human life and relationship become affirmed in a new way as the locus of God's relationship with God's people. The effect of this incarnational understanding of the one flesh tradition of Genesis is to consecrate it still further. God does not shun or disparage human flesh and bodiliness, but rather dwells within it. This reinforces the Genesis account that human life is in the image of God. While in the Genesis account, the man and woman became ashamed at their bodiliness, in John's gospel that bodiliness has been reclaimed as the place of God's dwelling. It is good!

The New Testament account, first from Jesus and then from Paul and John, thus has added to (not deleted from) the above list from Genesis, the following aspects to a covenantal relationship:

- the companionship of woman and man in marriage is not to be abused,
- the companionship of one body is a unity of one spirit,
- the one spirit of companionship requires ultimate mutuality and respect of the one to the other,
- God indwells in humanity, in such a way that human relationships themselves may be a sign of God's presence in the world.

What are the values in this which might pose a challenge to the proposal of surrogate motherhood? They would seem to be:

- the companionship of woman and man in married relationship is not to be disrespected;
- the relationship of woman and man itself may be a sign of God's presence;
- the one body nature of companionship requires ultimate mutuality and respect of the one to the other;
- humans are not only understood as in the image of God, but are also incarnated with the "flesh" of God (the Word).

The Ancient Traditions Incorporated: Our Covenant of Marriage

For comparison's sake, it is useful to shift ahead to the theology of Christians living years subsequent to these stories, to see how our particular church utilized the inherited traditions of this covenant of marriage. In the first Canadian Prayer Book of 1918, and then later of 1959, its statement of purpose (preface) to be read before the service explains,

> Matrimony; which is an honourable estate, instituted of God in the time of man's innocency, signifying unto us the mystical union that is betwixt Christ and his Church . . . was ordained for the hallowing of the union betwixt man and woman; for the procreation of children to be brought up in the fear and nurture of the Lord; and for the mutual society, help, and comfort, that the one ought to have of the other, in both prosperity and adversity.[2]

We can see that the Prayer Book is well aware, in these words, of the sense of covenant between man, woman, and God in this relationship it calls matrimonial. It sets out the covenantal pledges and expectations that are to be fulfilled, the primary pledge being the relationship of love:

> I, N. take thee N. to be my wedded wife/husband, to have and to hold from this day forward, for better for worse, for richer for poorer, in sickness and in health, to love and to cherish,

till death do us part, according to God's holy ordinance; and thereto I give thee my troth.[3]

Following the biblical traditions, it affirms that there is a foundational goodness to this union, including its sexual companionship, which involves no shame, as is indicated by the pledge taken with the exchange of rings:

With this ring I thee wed, with my body I thee honour, and all my worldly goods with thee I share.[4]

These words have been revised to make them more contemporary and clear as the English church gradually became the Anglican communion throughout the world, but the content of the words has not changed. The purpose of marriage, now in Canada using the more familiar term of *gift* for *blessing*, remains the same as the older English version cited above:

Marriage is a gift of God and a means of his grace, in which man and woman become one flesh. It is God's purpose that, as husband and wife give themselves to each other in love, they shall grow together and be united in that love, as Christ is united with his Church.

The union of man and woman in heart, body, and mind is intended for their mutual comfort and help, that they may know each other with delight and tenderness in acts of love [and that they may be blessed in the procreation, care, and upbringing of children].

In marriage, husband and wife give themselves to each other, to care for each other in good times and in bad. They are linked to each other's families, and they begin a new life together in the community.

It is a way of life that all should reverence, and none should lightly undertake.[5]

The values of the ancient Genesis story remain still intact, with the primary intention of the union to be for the mutual love, the "help and comfort" of the one to the other, that the relationship blesses the sexual intimacy of the couple ("delight and tenderness in acts of love"), that the union may bring with it the gift of procreation and upbringing of children, and that the created family is to be transformed into a procreating family. That this is, above all, a covenant of blessing is recalled in the blessing of rings for the pledge:

> Bless this ring given and received
> that it may be a symbol of the vow and covenant
> N. and N. have made this day.[6]

These services reflect the insights consolidated by the Anglican Church of Canada in its *Canon XXI—On Marriage in the Church*.[7] In the preface on the purpose of marriage it is affirmed that "marriage is a lifelong union in faithful love, for better or for worse, to the exclusion of all others on either side. This union is established by God's grace."

What is critical to note here is the sense of an absolute union (i.e., the tradition of one flesh) actually being established by God's grace. The purposes of marriage follow the priorities stated in the services themselves:

- mutual fellowship, support, and comfort,
- the procreation (if it may be) and nurture of children,
- the creation of a relationship in which sexuality may serve personal fulfilment in a community of faithful love.

Explicitly following and mentioning Genesis 1:27-31, the canon states, "The Church affirms in like manner the goodness of the union of man and woman in marriage, this being God's creation." Sensitive to the way previous generations may have lost the mutuality (and equality) of women and men, the marriage canon stresses "a new standard of reciprocal love between husband and wife was introduced leading towards an understanding of their equality" (I Cor. 7:3ff., 11:11ff., Eph. 5:21-33, Gal. 3:28).

The preface to the canon concludes by making quite clear that despite the church being set in different cultures and in contact with different systems of law, it is the "Christian standard of marriage" which is to be maintained — and the canon then deals with the regulations for such marriage as identified by the preface. In other words, the church does not understand itself as acting for the state in providing ways for persons to marry; it rather sees itself as promoting a distinctive Christian married state which is rooted in the Judeo-Christian tradition and enriched by deeper insights into companionship (love) coming from the tradition of Jesus.

So what, in conclusion, are the incorporated values of the Anglican Church of Canada from the Judeo-Christian tradition which might pose a challenge to a proposal such as surrogate motherhood? The central values would seem to be:

- the union of woman and man in marriage is a gift established by God's grace;
- the primary purpose of marriage is the support and comfort of the relationship in heart, body, and mind;
- sexual intimacy is a gift of the relationship itself;
- procreation of children is a further possible gift to the relationship.

From Experience: The Longing for Human Relatedness

Theology can be done in several ways. The most common is what we have done above: to look at the Hebrew and Christian traditions as sources for our understanding of who we have been and therefore who we ought to be. But there can be another starting-point: human living as we experience it today. This is the route of "theological anthropology," and it assumes that there is something revelatory which can be learned from being human itself (the human being becoming critically self-conscious of him/herself). But such learning from being human is done only because the theology of the Christian tradition affirms that this is, in fact, possible.

Theologically, the greatest support for such learning is found in the creation stories we have explored and find subsequently affirmed throughout the tradition: humankind is created in the image of God and God enters humanity as the Word made flesh. As such, human nature carries at its very best a reflection of God's nature, and therefore human nature itself is a source for knowledge of the intention and purpose of God for human living. The second major support for this learning comes through the understood transformative act of God in Christ, by which we understand our living to be animated by the Holy Spirit of God: "God's love has been poured into our hearts through the Holy Spirit which has been given to us" (Rom. 5:5).

Yet we will doubtless find a tension in human nature, for, as was seen in the creation stories and ever since, it is possible not to do as God would have us do. But God in Christ through the gift of the Holy Spirit enables us to retrieve our original image of God in a new way. As we look for this Holy Spirit in the human spirit, we must look for the points of tension between what seems towards God and what seems against God.

Two recent philosophers, Martin Buber and Gabriel Marcel,[8] try to follow the phenomenon of how the human spirit acts, and find ultimate significance in the reach or encounter one person has for another. The sense of isolation and aloneness of each individual is contrasted to a much deeper human yearning. They suggest that the finding of a deep fulfilment to one's own longing, through the discovery of another human spirit, is perhaps the most profound and self-evident "fact" of human living. Buber calls it the discovery of the "I-Thou" nature of human relationship, the reverence for a call to transcend one's own limited sphere of concerns as one person, in the discovery of a far greater value in living for a larger sphere of experience which we share with others. Marcel suggests further that the primary experience of being human is not the discovery of another "I," but of a "we." There is a mysterious but identifiable moment when our interest in ourself is subjugated by a far deeper interest for another. This happens between all persons—children, men, women—and when it happens, we notice that we take the other person's concerns to heart first. We instinctively protect the child, we instinctively support the friend, we instinctively cherish the lover. Canadian theologian Bernard Lonergan found the English phrase to "fall in love" an appropriate way to describe this instinctive attraction towards others which catapults an individual into a state of "being in love" with another person, or group, or even with God.[9] Love activates the affirmation of another person as a deeper end in itself than oneself. Happiness shifts from an individual to a desired shared experience. As happiness, interest, and concern shift from the self to the other, a new quality—vulnerability—shows itself. As one looks to the other, one gives up or surrenders the preoccupation of looking to oneself. But with that goes the hope, the yearning, that the other will in some way take up that love, and love one's own self in a way that mere self-love could not do. In a sense, once one has given oneself in a love towards some other(s), the self can only be found by being given back in affirmation and love. This becomes ultimate fulfilment in love: a unity and mutuality that finds the self not lost but gained through love of another/others. This discovery of the twofold movement of love is actually not dissimilar to the teaching of the Judeo-Christian tradition: the love of neighbour and of self are complementary and necessary to each other.

But there is a tension in this loving of the human spirit that would choose in fear or security to withdraw from the loving. The limited affirmation of self by the self may seem less risky than affirmation by others, and hence may be chosen. But in order for this scenario to work, possible affirmation of one self by other selves (i.e., to be loved!) must be ruled out and kept out. In identifying this movement of the spirit, Buber described it as the creation of the "I—it" relationship: detachment and objectification of the world and all other selves. This habitual way of viewing the world ultimately centres on oneself and a sense of hostility or anger towards the world/other people — for in a sense the world is resented for not sufficiently affirming one's primary sense of self. Out of fear or rejection, one sometimes stops or reverses one's natural development.

Where in all of this, then, might lie the sexual differentiation of woman from man? Is the transcending love for others found here? What is the role of the physical self and the body? The French philosopher Merleau-Ponty suggests that the experience of our bodies is absolutely key: it defines where me is and where it is not. All that I am is mediated through my body, and my spirit is not something detached from it. One cannot in fact think of another person without thinking (and feeling) the particularity of their actions, their gestures, their words said — and how each, in a physical sense, communicated through these things. If any of this is so, how much more must be the communication of physical intimacy between two persons!

Yet if sexual love is much like the affirmation of the other as we have described love itself, it is likely so attractive and yet threatening that one has to fall in love physically to discover it! From this insight come the various theories on the role of desire in sexual differentiation, and the uniqueness of sexual intercourse in being a profound physical and spiritual experience that cannot be experienced alone. To experience one flesh requires female and male. While self-gratification may be possible, the mutual fulfilment of two human beings in the act of love seems to have a transcending reality all of its own. Here the tension in human nature spoken of earlier reveals itself again; the sexual act can be a gratifier of self, or it can be a delight in the other. Through giving of oneself in the act, one can express love and delight in the other which, as it is returned, fulfills one's deepest yearnings. But if nothing is given in the act, then the gratification is merely one's own. Time enters in to attest to the significance of the giving. The more attentive and expressive the giving, the more it is remembered and longed for again. Love has a historical dimension; it evolves over time as opposed to being a mere random occurrence. As such, it longs for stability and continuance.

That sexual love can result in the conception and birth of a child is indeed awesome. The child as foetus is an obvious extension of the loved and beloved. Hence before its birth and the development of its own personality, a child has the projected personality of its parents — and is already loved and valued! Women talk of the experience of knowing and loving a child in the womb (bonding), say that each pregnancy and experience of the foetus is different—each almost has a personality of its own. Hence by the time of birth, a deep bond has already formed between mother and child entirely through sense and feel. The intimacy of nursing upon birth is another deeply physical and spiritual experience, one that some women describe as having associations of the pleasurable intimacy of the act of love. The father of the child has less obvious forms of interaction with the child, yet most fathers would describe a bonding occurring as they hold, cuddle, and feel their child. In this surrounding of projected and extended love, the human child emerges, helpless itself for two to three years. There seems to be an obvious link between the generation and projection of love and care in the relationship of a woman and man, and the protection and nurture of the child conceived in that love.

How do these reflections relate to our questions concerning surrogate motherhood? They seem to provide us with another kind of evidence for some basic human values not unlike those we traced from the biblical tradition. These human values seem to be:

- there is a primary discovery and valuing of another human being, a "thou," in human relationship;
- in the experience of responding to another, one's own deeper sense of identity is found;
- the body and sexual intimacy give profound expression to the relationship of love;
- the committed and mutual love of intimate sexual relationship provides a prior love and commitment for a child who may be born into that relationship.

Another Tradition: Accepting Human Limits

One other theme that we need to recollect in order to discuss a new proposal such as surrogate motherhood is the tradition of human limitation: what humans do/should not do. We met this in the Genesis creation story in the significance of the tree of knowledge which humans could reach, but were not supposed to touch. It is important to note that the first "sin" of the humans in the garden was to exceed that limit. But there is a long theological tradition of human excesses, particularly in relation to God. One of the oldest versions goes back to the memory of the Mosaic covenant of Sinai. In Exodus 20:3, the Decalogue (Ten Commandments) begins, "You shall have no other gods before me." The first four commandments are expressions of the zeal and holiness of God: that apart from Yahweh, there is no other, and therefore no image shall be worshipped, God's name shall never be taken in vain, and the sabbath day of God shall always be kept. These commandments effectively define the region of the holy of God, in awareness, representation, language, and deference. And holy things — like the Ark — are untouchable (II Sam. 6:6), not to be looked upon (Num. 4:18), not to be encroached upon.

But like the Genesis story of the tree of good and evil, this otherness is within the experience of humankind, while at the same time beyond the experience of humankind. Holiness is to be realized and respected ("all the earth shall be filled with the glory of God" Num. 14:21), but that glory is not to be encroached upon. This is the "zeal" of Yahweh (Ex. 10:5, 34:14, Deut. 6:14) which is the expression of holiness, yet which cannot be measured or discovered by any human standard.

But in contrast, humans are limited and weak alongside of God:

> He does not faint or grow weary,
> his understanding is unsearchable.
> He gives power to the faint,
> and to him who has no might
> he increases strength.
> Even youths shall faint and be weary
> and young men shall fall exhausted. (Is. 40:28-31)

The capacities of the body, such as strength and energy, are a key form of limitation that humans must accept. Also limited are the functions of the body; God needs no sleep as does the human (Ps. 121:4), God sees differently than do humans (Job 10:4), and can know the secrets of the heart (Ps. 139:23). The zeal or glory of God illustrates human limitation by comparison.

Set in the creation stories of Genesis there is the unique story of the Tower of Babel. In that story of the building of a city in the plain is imaged the development of civilization, and economic and political organizations. The ambitious will to greatness built on human potential is expressed in the words:

> Come, let us build ourselves a city
> and a tower with its top in the heavens
> and let us make a name for ourselves. (Gen. 11:4)

The use of the material of creation (earth and bitumen), its production into bricks and mortar, and its use to accomplish an exaggerated goal (a tower "with its top in the heavens"), to "make a name for ourselves," typify human refusal to be limited and instead desire to encroach on the holiness and zeal of God. The words ascribed to God thus refer to far more than this mere primeval tower:

> This is only the beginning of what they will do
> and nothing that they propose to do
> will now be impossible for them. (Gen. 11:6)

As with the tree of good and evil, it is within reach of the humans, but God advises its being beyond humanity's use. In this story, the judgment of God condemns this project and all similar human projects. Of necessity, they "left off building the city." There is no grace or reprieve in this story; the limit was exceeded. This experience becomes a legacy for subsequent human potential and creativity, which is itself a God-given gift that has made the human a "little lower than the angels" (Ps. 8:3). But its bounds can be overstepped. The story suggests that space between God and the human has to be respected.

The story of the tower helps us reflect on a more current picture of being human in the world. Limitations constantly appear, especially when we have something else in mind. As this paper is being written, the Soviet Union is reeling from an earthquake in Armenia at the very time that the nation has set a major political reform of *glasnost* (openness) and *perestroika* (restructuring) as its national goal. This impressive goal has had some unforeseen limitations. The decade of the eighties has seen tremendous advances in medical science such as cancer and heart therapies, only to be stymied by an entirely new threat to life: AIDS. Human medicine is not capable of overall guarantees to health: only particular gains seem possible. On a more personal level, young couples re-arrange their lives to accommodate the careers of both, only to find that their timetable of having a child at age 35 did not take into account a prevalent difficulty in conception. Childbearing is not reducible to mere planning and production. In particular areas, humans seem capable of some very exceptional things, only to find out that some other and uncontrollable factor prevents them. Certitude in knowledge, in science, and in human affairs always seems elusive and tenuous.

Here the significance of the Genesis tree symbol of good and evil perhaps enters in, because by that story humankind supposedly now has this discerning capacity. So what is a good? Is it whatever is good for me (an individual), or is it what is good for the world in which I live (the community)? Can we discern in a situation a movement towards God or against God? In the Babylon story, we witness a tower being built which only benefits the zeal of rulers who wish to make a name for themselves. But what of the builders, and what of their society? Did the tower ensure a good water supply, safe roads, and sufficient food for all — or did the tower siphon off those benefits so that all energies and resources could be put to its building? If the tower produced those ills, then how could it be seen as a good? By comparison, the tower emerges as more of a source of evil than good. It neither benefits the society around it, nor does it give any more benefit to the rulers than boost their own self-image.

In terms of our discussion of a proposal for surrogate motherhood, how does this tradition of human limitation apply? It would urge a basic caution in moving beyond a well-defined limit from the wisdom of our past — such as, in this case, the acceptance of the regular limits to the capacity of human fertility which any married couple would normally encounter. That might serve as a base line to the discussion. To use a new technology or social practice to go beyond that limit calls for some discernment of good and evil. If a couple may be enabled to have a genetically related child (an individual good), what will be the effect on the world around them — for example, the woman who actually bears the child, the child itself who was removed from its birthing mother, or the society which no longer needs to connect actual birthing with the deeply seated sense of responsibility to parent? In extending human freedom to this degree, have we neglected other deeper God-given human obligations which are actually at stake here? Is this extension of human activity beyond the normal limits of human capacity, a good for both the individual and the world around us, or will it produce in the end a greater evil? Are we exceeding the limits of human capacity and entering a field more capably known by God? What do we discern?

This tradition of limitation, therefore, leaves us with:

- awareness that the human condition is, by definition, limited;
- there is activity within and beyond that limit which presumes a greater capacity than we have (God);
- in perceiving an appropriate limit to human activity, we must look for discernment as to the good and evil which such action could create.

Integrating and Applying the Traditions: Surrogate Motherhood

Surrogate motherhood, as a proposed social practice, represents both the old and the new in terms of a remedy for a couple's infertility. It is as old as the Genesis story of Hagar, the slave girl of supposedly infertile Sarah, who bore Abraham the subsequently rejected son Ishmael (Gen. 16 ff.). The infertility was remedied, but the relationship of love and parenting proved hurtful and incapable of achieving the goals of the remedy. It is as new as combinations of therapeutic donor insemination (T.D.I.) and *in vitro* fertilization (I.V.F.), which can enable an infertile couple, whether husband or wife, to have a child genetically related (to one or possibly both of them), when carried and birthed by a surrogate mother, yet declared to be (but not in actuality) the child only of the arranging couple. As this new proposal is put alongside the heritage of values from the Judeo-Christian tradition, we would find grounds to respond that this surrogacy will very likely be unable to achieve its goal, and instead may be hurtful as well. In chapter 3 Phyllis Creighton has described the specific abuses, while in chapter 4 Marsha Hewitt has traced the destructive values present in this abuse. But from the point of view of a positive regard for the Judeo-Christian tradition, specifically what would lead us to a foundational questioning of this proposal of surrogacy?

Relationship, Sexual Intimacy, and Procreation of Children

The Judeo-Christian tradition, as rooted in the Genesis creation stories ("Origins of the Covenant") and subsequently affirmed in Christian scriptures ("the 'New' Covenant"), makes a link between a married relationship, sexual intimacy in relationship, and procreation of children from that relationship. Something transformative occurs when two "become one flesh." Jesus seems both to know of and to confirm the centrality of this insight. Paul uses it to explain the knowing intimacy between Christ and the church — the source of his ultimate analogy of relationship. These traditions become integrated in the church's understanding of marriage which teaches that the primary purpose of marriage is the "lifelong union of faithful love" ("The Ancient Traditions").

Looking at the same phenomenon from the perspective of

human experience. ("From Experience"), we found a surprising correspondence in the "I—Thou" relationship of mutuality that happens to people when they "fall in love." The self, discovered through the affirmation of another, longs for permanency in relationship, and the sexual intimacy it provides is a vehicle for expression of meaning between two persons. In the context of this commitment, a child can be conceived and born — to be set in an already prior context of commitment. There seem to be both external (the tradition) and internal (the phenomenon) reasons why married relationship, sexual intimacy, and procreation are set together. But the proposal of surrogacy seems to remove the relationship of some of these elements — particularly sexual intimacy and procreation. What effect then would the necessary clinical procedures have upon the contracting parents and the birth mother, as the means of procreation, and upon the children? Who is benefited by having a genetically related child (although it may not be related to both "parents," depending on the intention in acquiring a child) as opposed to say, an adopted child? More important still, what effect does this practice have on the birthing surrogate mother, who must have the experience of bonding with the child in her womb, to which most women attest? Given the nature of the integration of married relationship, sexual intimacy, and procreation, it would seem a very serious and likely hurtful thing indeed to propose the dismantling of what in both tradition and experience are integrally related phenomena.

"Surrogate" Marriages, Their Children, and the Mother of Birth
Particularly then, we must ask whether the proposal of surrogacy would suggest a shifting of the nature of Christian marriage. In the sections above, we have seen how, from the biblical traditions through to their current application in the covenant of marriage ("The Ancient Traditions"), the primary purpose of marriage is "a union of faithful love" and not the procreation of children. In fact, the marriage service directly alludes to procreation "if it may be" and the nurture of children ("The Ancient Traditions"). Infertility has never been grounds to declare a marriage invalid (although royal families have certainly tried to make it so and have, in some cases, succeeded), and yet that problem has always been common enough to warrant its clarification in the service itself. Yet does the inability to procreate a child make

a couple's union less than complete, less than the sacrament of unity? Does it deny a couple the willingness to share their love with others, or remove a couple from the opportunity to nurture a child, to which the age-old tradition of adoption attests? What can be learned from that tradition? Perhaps the most useful insight is that almost all legal and social considerations of the practice of adoption focus on the child and not on the receiving couple. For whatever the reasons a child is without support of its birthing parents, the first consideration is the child's well-being in the care of another set of parents. In a less than ideal situation, the child is freely given love and support. This is not an early custom intended to address a couple's inability to conceive children, although it may happen to provide for a childless couple. It is an arrangement to care for a child.

Most civil jurisdictions have learned from these adopted children of their need to identify their birthing parents, and most now provide such a means upon the adopted child reaching an adult age. The search is always for the birth mother. It would seem that not only does a mother bond to her child in the womb, but in some elemental way the child also bonds with its mother. A recent study of adoption and birth-parent reunions says:

> For a human being who has been unnaturally separated from his/her origins, the reunion with the birth parent is an integral event in his/her life. . . . The reunion provides a bridge to the adoptee's beginnings and answers questions about the past and present. Whether the outcome of the reunion fulfills fantasies is not so important as the fact that it gives the adoptee, finally, a feeling of wholeness.[10]

Surrogacy would produce this same search, but will the role of the birthing mother remain as central to the event as the supposed donors of sperm and ovum? Would her role as the actual mother be now erased by law? And further, what has the separation of conception, pregnancy, and birthing into multiple parts, dependent upon medical technology, done to the wholeness of a child's origination and upbringing within an identifiable family? What is the child to be told? This disintegration of wholeness and continuity in the conception, birthing, and parenting of children surely would destroy a meaningful integration of these three things, with likely some very painful results for children, birthing mothers, parents, and society as a whole.

Infertility, Limitation, and the Marriage
In this proposal of surrogacy, what concern has been extended to infertile couples who, by the time they may consider some form of surrogacy arrangements, will already have gone through several years of consultation with infertility clinics and also will very likely have explored local adoption procedures? They will already have a strain on their marriage relationship since one and possibly both will have discovered he or she is "the problem." They will have discovered that adoption may involve a wait of over five years, with no guarantee that a child will be placed with them, or that they will have any degree of choice about the child offered. Theologically, is this not the point where some awareness of human limitation, however painful, has to take place? ("Another Tradition"). There are several aspects to this caution, and surely the first is the concern for a couple's marriage. However much one or the other partner may wish a child, will the generation of a child outside that couple's intimacy help or hinder their relationship? Is a couple less than a whole relationship without children? Then further, some couples talk about a right to have a child, but has such a right ever been the case? One may have a right to marry, but does that translate into reciprocity, a right to a marriage? Surely it needs the willingness of another person, and that cannot be guaranteed or purchased! In a similar way, might not our proposed fertility as a couple need the actual consent (capacity) of our bodies, which just might not be present for whatever reason? Does that situation release us from paying attention to long-standing Jewish and Christian wisdom for the integration of married relationships, sexual intimacy, and procreation as the means within which to realize the hope of children? Beyond that, do we have the right to generate life outside our own human means and limitations? At such points of human limitation we are supposedly given the means of discerning where to see good or evil ("A Method for Reflecting" and "From Experience"). Does our wish for an individual child (my child) balance the possible negative effects upon an actual child and upon others who will be affected by their proximity to this choice of ours, to say nothing of the possibly devastating effect on our

marriage itself? As the tenor of this section indicates, we see an accumulation of likely negative effects to far outweigh what might be gained for any couple's individual good.

The Sacrament of One Flesh and One Spirit

In our recovery of the New Testament tradition, we discovered not only the affirmation of the Genesis tradition of one flesh, but also the understanding by which the married relationship represents such a discovery of oneness that Paul kept proposing it as a way to describe the intimacy of Christ and the church. This unity in relationship is a human metaphor for perceiving the unity that is possible for us with God. The traditions of the church have so affirmed this insight that the more Catholic traditions would call marriage sacramental, as does our Anglican Church of Canada: "marriage is a gift of God and a means of his grace" ("The Ancient Traditions"). If this is so, what would it mean to remove from that sacramentality a central part of the gift, which is sexual intimacy and its context for the procreation of children? Would this not have an effect upon the "means of grace" of the relationship? In "From Experience" we have traced the dynamics of the human spirit as being able to enter into a vulnerable self-giving in which the self became discovered through being gifted to another. Is this something of the mystery of this relationship of unity that Paul was referring to between Christ and the church ("The 'New' Covenant")? Have we weighed our difficulty in having a child against the giftedness of our relationship which surrogacy procedures could destroy? While we may understand procedures to overcome human infertility, are we equally knowledgeable about the sacramentality of marriage itself which we could be bypassing? If we as a couple can have children, as long as we use another man's sperm, another woman's ovum and womb, have we realized the gift of children in the mutual self-giving of our marriage — or have we simply arranged to birth a child in some way physically related to one of us? What might we have achieved compared with what we might have lost?

Thou, It, and the Image of God

One of the beautiful ways the Genesis story images a married relationship is the way a child leaves father and mother and becomes one flesh in a totally new relationship. It is an image of new origination. Two persons discover in each other a "Thou," another human spirit whose significance transcends the importance of one's own self. Of all human experiences, this most enables one to recognize something beyond one's own body as being of infinite worth and value. The Judeo-Christian tradition calls it image of God ("Origins of the Covenant" and "The 'New' Covenant"). But before that discovery, as Buber suggested, another human being can seem a mere body, an object, an "it." Does the proposal of surrogacy not make some involved in that arrangement mere objects, an "it"? What is done to the mother of birth, whether she has or has not supplied the ovum for the conception? Does she not bond with the child, as any other mother would? Does the child not bond with her? Yet they will be separated at birth, for supposedly a prior relationship. Can anything be more prior than a birth? Surely such a social arrangement not only disguises the real relationships, but thereby renders both mother and child an "it". Not only does the situation abuse them, it also reduces the intended mother and father to objects in this relationship. Having compromised their own relationship, how able are they to provide a relationship of gifted love for the nurture of their own developed and adopted child? Have we packaged the gift of the image of God, the thou of our human experience, rendering it a mere "it," a thing?

Conclusion

The theological traditions of the Judeo-Christian heritage are so diverse and layered that they seldom are able to provide clear answers, yes or no, to new situations, new technologies, new practices. Their contribution is not foresight into the future, but rather insight from faithful living in the past. In this case, the heritage reminds us that the marriage of a woman and a man into one flesh is not for the production of children, but for the unity of a man and a woman just as God desires the unity of God with humankind. The first gift is this self-giving relationship. An added gift is the children thus made possible. Human science might make more things possible. While human science can produce cells as well as objects, it cannot produce relationships. And a loving relationship is the place for a new relationship to grow: a child of a family. No social or medical procedure should ask of that couple anything which would compromise their relationship. No couple should ask of themselves what would lessen their relationship. No child should be burdened with subsequent relationship that may be tenuous at best or hurtful at worst. No mother should have the significance of her birthing lessened by being labelled "surrogate." Too many values and persons seem capable of being hurt or abused in such an arrangement to warrant either experimenting or proceeding with it.

What then is a childless couple to do in this age of new technologies and practices which address infertility? Perhaps the first thing our church can do is affirm the relationship of the couples themselves as the primary gift of their marriage. Like any gift, such relationships need to be held up and appreciated by their communities. Few individuals enter a relationship simply to have children; the relationship itself is the gift. But children are a not inappropriate wish of any couple; the gift of further life to a relationship of two lives is a deeply spiritual hope that out of a union may come a new origination. No one, especially our church, should put down such a generous hope.

There will always be a need for adopted parents of children who cannot be with the parents of their birth. But beyond that, our parish and neighbourhood communities can become places for extended families, in which the whole community benefits from the gift of children and new life. Couples are not the only ones to need such a presence.

On more of a moral level, our church can contribute to the society around it centuries of wisdom concerning the meaning and value of married relationship — while also encouraging modern technological society to reflect on what might be some limits to human proposal and experimentation. The past three centuries have witnessed profound advances in our technological and industrial capacity. We have found both amazing ways to protect and encourage life, as well as ways to infect and systematically destroy it. We can change organs, change sexes, and have even tried to change races. But have we equally tried to protect relationships, cherish intimacy, support bonding, and enable the self-surrender of union in the one flesh? Our technological advances encourage us to overlook what may be basic human limitations (what may be detrimental and hurtful) by considering instead attractive human possibilities. By looking at the quality or value in any proposal, as well as its possible hurtfulness, we may be enabled to discern what may be good or evil in the garden of our world. In the proposal of surrogate motherhood, we have found central values of the Judeo-Christian tradition ignored, as well as other implications which could be hurtful or damaging. While we pledge our support to couples who would wish to have children from their union but find themselves unable to do so, we would not recommend for them, or for the society which we hold in common, either a practice or an experimentation with what has been termed a proposal for surrogate motherhood.

Notes

1. For a detailed study of these texts, *see* Phyllis Trible, *God and the Rhetoric of Sexuality* (Philadelphia: Fortress Press, 1978). A good summary can be found in Judy Rois, *Joint Heirs of the Grace of Life*. (Toronto: Doctrine and Worship Committee of the Anglican Church of Canada, 1987.)
2. This passage can be found in *The Book of Common Prayer*, (Toronto: Oxford University Press, 1959), p.564.
3. *Book of Common Prayer*, p.566.
4. *Book of Common Prayer*, p.566.
5. *The Book of Alternative Services of the Anglican Church of Canada*. (Toronto: Anglican Book Centre, 1985), p.528-29.
6. *Book of Alternative Services*, p.532.
7. *Handbook of General Synod of the Anglican Church of Canada*, 7th ed (Toronto: Anglican Book Centre, 1984), p.99.
8. A good overview of their thought and others mentioned below can be found in John Macqarrie, *Twentieth-Century Religious Thought* (New York: Harper and Row, 1963).
9. Bernard Lonergan, *Method in Theology* (New York: Herder and Herder, 1972), pp.33, 36, 105-6, 240.
10. Arthur Sorosky, Annette Baren, and Reuben Pannor, *The Adoption Triangle* (New York: Doubleday, 1984), p.157.

Surrogate Parenting — Legal Aspects

Bruce Alton

Introduction

Surrogate parenting uses modern reproductive technology, but it is more importantly a social issue which raises questions of a much broader scope than those of medical ethics. It is an agreement or contract to use medical technology in such a way that a woman produces and transfers custody of a child to a man and his wife. Whether set forth in a written contract or not, such an arrangement between people is subject to legal analysis, not least because it can become a matter of legal dispute.

Should the law permit such agreements and, if so, subject to what regulations? Should the law ban surrogate parenting? Why? And how could it do so most effectively? Are all surrogate parenting agreements questionable, or only those involving payment? There is currently no clear consensus on such matters in Canada; we must ask why.

Canada in the late twentieth century is officially (and increasingly in fact) a multicultural and religiously pluralistic society. It does not follow that the law must try to accommodate all moral viewpoints. But the question whether, and how, recourse to law should be a means to social and moral control is much more complex than it once was.[1]

In addition, at the time of writing there are uncertainties which arise from the inclusion of "freedom of religion and conscience" in the Canadian Charter of Rights (section 2 [a]) and how this might be interpreted on the subject of surrogate parenting, especially the non-commercial — altruistic — variety, by the courts. As well, it is unclear whether the Canada/U.S. Free Trade Agreement would permit a commercialization of surrogacy as a "service industry" in Canada on the grounds that, in a few case decisions, it seems to have been so deemed in the United States.[2]

The view of this task force is that Anglicans have sound theological and moral grounds for rejecting surrogate parenting as a way of "solving," should they face it, the painful fact of infertility. We also maintain that there are sound reasons to try to ensure that surrogate parenting, if it cannot be eliminated from our society, be so constrained by law as to protect prospective birth mothers from exploitation, to serve the best interests of children so brought into being, and to ban commercialization of the procedure.

In thus recommending against surrogate parenting to our family of faith, and indeed to all Canadians, we are aware that some may sincerely disagree. To those people we say that, at the very least, if they intend to engage in the practice or advise others on the matter, they should be aware that surrogate parenting arrangements may even now (without legislative changes which we recommend for study) be illegal in Canada. There is wide difference of legal opinion on the matter, but the preponderance of opinion seems to be that under Canadian provincial laws as they now stand, surrogate parenting is a potential legal nightmare for those who contemplate it.

To those who agree with our conclusions, we would add that we all have a duty to inform ourselves about present legal aspects of the issue before we act individually or collectively in any attempt to influence legislation. Factual analysis of the law must come before legal change.

Since adoption law is a matter of provincial jurisdiction, legal aspects of surrogate parenting are not uniform in Canada, and they are a matter of some dispute as well within the legal profession and by informed legislators. We caution our readers that in what follows we can provide only a very general analysis which is subject to jurisdictional variation and conflicting interpretation.

A World View

First, it is useful to try to put the legal aspects of surrogate parenting in something of a world perspective.

There is little evidence to suggest that at the present time surrogate mothering (or, for that matter, artificial means of reproduction) is a priority issue in other than first world countries which have a low birth rate and a rather delayed age for first pregnancies.

Commercial surrogacy arrangements are generally sought by

the affluent with birth mothers who are (relatively) poor, usually within the same country. One reason for a lack of international "trade" is the complexity of law on the matter; international adoptions are complicated enough. But it should be noted that legislation against surrogacy, or even legislation permitting non-commercial agreements, could make third world peoples vulnerable, as it has in the case of adoption, to those who can afford to go outside their country in an "easy" search of their goal.

Affluent Western countries which have tried to come to terms with surrogate parenting have generated more than fifteen major reports by special government-commissioned or other influential bodies,[3] most of which conclude that the practice is unacceptable. Canadians might note that only the report of the Ontario Law Reform Commission and that of the Dutch Health Council conclude that both commercial and non-commercial forms of surrogate parenting are acceptable in principle (that is, if subject to regulatory control).[4]

Attention should also be drawn to the Warnock Committee report in Britain[5] which concluded that "regulation" of the practice would in fact encourage it. It recommended to the government the criminalization of all surrogate agencies, profit and non-profit, and the passage of statutes making all surrogacy contracts unenforceable in the courts; but it stopped short of recommending that private surrogate arrangements should be criminalized. Another report, of the British Council for Science and Society, had earlier expressed approval of non-commercial surrogacy. The British parliament enacted the Surrogacy Arrangements Act in July 1985, which attempts to prevent third parties from deriving financial gain from surrogacy. It is inaccurate to say that the British law in itself outlaws commercial surrogacy, but adoption law in Britain prohibits payment for an adopted child and thus, together, the laws have this effect. "To date, however, voluntary surrogacy is not illegal in Britain."[6]

A year earlier, the state of Victoria in Australia enacted The Infertility (Medical Procedures) Act after a series of major studies.[7] By this legislation, it is an offence to give or receive payment in a surrogacy arrangement, advertising of any kind is forbidden, and surrogate contracts of all kinds are void. "Altruistic volunteer" surrogacy of a private nature would not however be illegal.[8] This legal stand is perhaps the most firm and decisive one internationally.

The situation in the United States and Canada is rather different, in part because commercial surrogate mothering has already established a foothold in the U.S., and in part because the more influential studies have been done by groups focusing rather narrowly on the matter of contracts, no doubt because of cases (such as Baby M) of disputed custody of babies born of a surrogate parenting agreement. But not all North American studies slant toward a presumption of the legitimacy of surrogate parenting contracts. An important exception in Canada is the study of the Barreau du Québec, to which we will refer shortly.

The United States

When the New York State Task Force on Life and the Law examined U.S. state laws, they found that, as of September 1987, surrogate parenting bills had been introduced in 26 of the 50 states and the District of Columbia. The bills vary. Some call for regulation, some prohibit contracts, some simply call for further study. By March 1988, four states (Indiana, Kentucky, Louisiana, and Nebraska) had enacted legislation declaring contracts for surrogate parenting "void and unenforceable as against public policy"; two others (Arkansas and Nevada) recognized them as "enforceable, subject to judicial review." Legislation prohibiting surrogate parenting contracts was pending in other states, including New York.[9] After the New York report was published, Michigan has enacted the first U.S. state law making surrogacy contracts a felony, with penalties up to five years in jail and a $50,000 fine.

The New York study recommends permission of noncommercial surrogacy "similar to the way the New York State Legislature has addressed adoptions — by prohibiting payments to the mother of the child, to brokers and to others, except for medical and other necessary expenses."[10] The effect of such legislation would be to leave the decision entirely in the hands of the birthing mother, to block any monetary return for such action, and to deploy family and adoption law (rather than contract law, over which they have precedence) to this end, modifying them as necessary. We are in general agreement with this approach.

We cannot predict the outcome of legislative action in the other states of the United States. In some states, in the absence of legislation, commercial surrogacy by contract may continue and spread, though subject to litigation if any of the parties challenge the agreement. In other states, all contracting may be banned. In still others, contracts may be permitted (perhaps subject to judicial review) but without payment beyond medical and legal necessities.

Canada

As in the United States, family and adoption law is a provincial (state) prerogative. Two important studies and reports (in Ontario and Quebec) will be cited here. We are not aware of comparable studies in other provinces.

But first, it is important to note that commercial surrogate parenting does not appear to be widespread within Canada because it seems it would, if challenged by any party, run afoul of adoption laws prohibiting payment in any sense or at any stage of the process.

It does appear possible, though legally complicated, for a Canadian couple to arrange a surrogacy contract with an American woman, or for an American couple to do so with a Canadian woman, provided the adoption of the child is by private (and undisputed) arrangement within a jurisdiction which does not bar payment in such cases. Whether a contract in such cases would hold up in court in the case of a custody dispute would depend on the jurisdiction; opinion is widespread that in Canadian jurisdictions it would not, again because of generally tougher adoption laws.

The main reason, then, for commercial surrogate parenting not spreading rapidly in Canada is the stringency of provincial legislation against "buying," or even appearing to buy, babies. This point deserves elaboration in understanding the Canadian situation.

While legal disputes may arise around the so-called contract, they will most likely do so at the time of, or with respect to, transfer of custody by adoption. But there is an important difference between ordinary adoption and adoption in the case of surrogate parenting. The essential feature of surrogate parenting is that the birthing mother freely and consciously intends *not* to act as a custodial parent of the child to whom she gives birth, past the date upon which she transfers custody. In other words, she bears the child for the express purpose of handing her/him over to others. That, at least, is her intent when she undertakes the arrangement; that she might change her mind is a large part of the problem (from a legal-contract perspective).

Two other aspects of the matter should be noted. First, it is commonly argued that in a surrogacy arrangement birthing is a service provided for another person or persons, and that the legal intention (transfer of custody of the child) is very much of secondary importance. Perhaps for this reason the Ontario Law Reform Commission, while it argues that "it is this transfer of custody, with the parental rights and responsibilities incident thereto, that lies at the heart of the surrogate motherhood controversy,"[11] holds nevertheless that the matter cannot be simply *reduced* to an adoption model. It is true that transfer of custody is but the final and formal stage in a whole process undertaken for the purported benefit of the custodial parents-to-be; that is why we prefer to refer to them as the surrogates.

Nevertheless, we need also to point out again that neither is surrogate parenting a mere incubational process or a mere medical technology, even though surrogate mothering in the modern context[12] entails artificial reproductive interventions. Giving birth is a human procreative act which might be thought of (whatever the social, marital, or contractual involvement of others) as a service of the woman primarily to the child in her womb. She alone of our species is capable of this service and she, in the final analysis, bears both the responsibility and the privilege of deciding whether, and how, that service will be delivered to the child. Thus in our view contract to others, and a desire to help the infertile, are superseded by the mother's primary relation to the child of her womb. This view of the birth mother is enshrined in federal statute under the Vital Statistics Act: "There is a legal presumption, although rebuttable, that the child is the child of the [birthing] mother and her husband."[13]

The point we wish to stress here is the primacy of the birthing act over contract, agreement, intent to serve others, and intent to transfer custody. Giving birth is more than an action; it is undergirded by a relationship between the pregnant woman and her child. While others (including the state) may have legitimate interests and even a stake in the process, they may intrude upon that relationship only with just cause and with the onus of justification for intervention lying on them. The birthing mother's *prima facie* custody of, and responsibility for, the child is enshrined in law, in biological reality, and in Christian theology alike. Those who admit the importance of preserving the social order would do well to look to these roots of social stability before giving any precedence, contractual or not, to other persons.

For these reasons, agreements with other parties, even where the paternity of the genetic father is acknowledged implicitly or explicitly, and even in cases of *in vitro* fertilization where genetic maternity is acknowledged to be derived externally, do not alter the fact in law as well as in practice, that "a person is the child of his or her natural parents,"[14] and that by presumption the woman who gives birth is the maternal parent.

It is disputable whether, in common law, the genetic father of a child would have "an absolute right to custody of a legitimate child, even as against the natural mother."[15] Such an outdated view is giving way to judgments which serve the best interests of the child. In any case, it seems to many that this tradition could not, or should not, apply in the case of surrogate parenting on the grounds that the child is not legitimate. But the comparison of surrogate parenting with extra-marital infidelity, or prostitution, or adultery, does not lend itself to useful legal distinctions even though it may offer pause for moral reflection.

The more important matter, from a legal perspective, is that this common law tradition has been most widely interpreted as being grounded in the principle "that parental rights were not transferable," even by agreement, and that this judicial position "extended to mothers as well."[16] While this position is always a matter of judicial decision, and while in Canada there is a wider range of judicial opinion on the matter than in England, the application of the principle of the non-transferability of parental rights is still very widely maintained in law.[17] Exceptions are, of course, entertained; that is why case law is so important. But exceptions are always considered and *determined in terms of what is in the best interests of the child.*

According to the Ontario Law Reform Commission the present situation in Ontario, and as far as we can determine in the rest of Canada as well, is that

1. "except in the case of adoption, it is not possible at present to alter parentage or the status of a child";[18]

2. the child of a surrogate mother is *presumed* to be parented by his/her mother and her husband, if he exists;
3. the genetic father would have to "obtain a declaratory order of paternity and a custody order under the *Children's Law Reform Act*, having first obtained the agreement of the surrogate mother not to contest the order";[19]
4. this would have to be followed with proceedings toward stepparent adoption by the genetic father's spouse, again with consent obtained from the surrogate mother;
5. provincial legislation would prohibit any payment, or any agreement for payment, in relation to the adoption;[20]
6. finally, until the adoption order had been legally passed, the birthing mother's right to contest the proceedings, including custody, is indisputable; she can change her mind at any point.

It is important for participants in this process to note 1) that "the route just described is highly circuitous,"[21] 2) it is further constrained by adoption laws, and 3) it protects the birthing mother's right to reverse her choice, though not absolutely (the best interests of the child always being the decisive element) about transfer of custody right up to the final moment. In other words, while contract law has some weight if it comes to a court battle, the rights of the birthing mother, and the best interests of the child, appear to be the overriding legal determinants in Canada because surrogate parenting is essentially a matter of *adoption*.

The Ontario Law Reform Commission View

The Ontario Law Reform Commission majority argues, on the grounds that a ban might force the practice underground, that commercial and non-commercial surrogacy should be regulated, with extensive oversight by family law courts.

However well intentioned the O.L.R.C. recommendations for legal reform in these matters may be, we think they would promote surrogate parenting in Ontario and transform a very limited practice into a regulated but essentially dehumanizing experience, overburden an already greatly strained court system, and serve essentially only the legal machinery and lawyers.

We consider the thrust of the proposed legislation to be essentially wrong minded. We draw attention especially to the following items in the proposed regulatory scheme which would make such contracts both binding and inhumane for the mother:[22]

37. On the hearing of the application for approval of a surrogate motherhood arrangement, the court should be required to assess the suitability of the prospective parents for participation in such an arrangement.
42. . . . the court should be required to assess the suitability of the prospective surrogate mother.
49. *A child born* pursuant to an approved surrogate motherhood arrangement *should be surrendered immediately upon birth* to the social parents. Where a surrogate mother refuses to transfer the child, the court should order that the child be delivered to the social parents. In addition, where the court is satisfied that the surrogate mother intends to refuse to surrender the child upon birth, it should be empowered, prior to the birth of the child to make an order for transfer of custody upon birth.
51. Legislation should provide that *no payment be made* in relation to a surrogate motherhood arrangement *without the prior approval of the court.*
56. Upon the birth of a child pursuant to an approved surrogate motherhood arrangement, the social parents should be recognized as the parents of the child for all legal purposes, *and the surrogate mother should have no legal relationship to the child.*
59. The birth of a child pursuant to an approved surrogate motherhood arrangement should be registered under the *Vital Statistics Act*, showing the social parents as the mother and father. *The surrogate mother should not be named in the register of births*; nor should the fact that the child has been born to a surrogate mother appear in the register.

It could be, and is, argued that such provisions are intended to eliminate as much as possible "confusion of identity" problems for the child so born. But the effect on the mother, it must be seen at once, is inversely proportional: she would be, under such a regulatory scheme, nothing more than the paid baby-producer we have denounced, in other sections of this report, as decidedly sub-human and in violation of any religious or socially responsible view of human procreation.

The Barreau du Québec View

Quite at odds with the OLRC view, the Barreau du Québec has recommended in a recent report[23] that surrogate parenting not be accorded legal sanction. Finding none of the arguments in its favour to outweigh the costs of creating and using a child as a commodity to satisfy parenting desires, the view of the majority on the committee was that surrogate parenting contracts are contrary to public order, that sanctions within the Child Protection Act should be specifically extended to penalize intermediaries in such arrangements, and that the Civil Code should be amended to state that no preferential right of adoption should be accorded to the wife of the genetic father of a child. A minority view was that while intermediaries should be subject to penalty, the law should not prohibit arrangements of a purely private nature.

No legislative action has been taken to date on the report, but only minor changes in Quebec statute law would be necessary to effect the majority view.

Proposed Federal Legislation

On 24 February 1988 a private member's bill, Bill C-284, introduced by M.P. Sheila Copps, received first reading in parliament. The bill would amend the Criminal Code of Canada by penalizing profit-making on surrogacy arrangements by agencies or go-betweens, entering into surrogate parenting arrangements on a commercial basis, and advertising for women to become surrogate mothers. The bill died with the dissolution of the last parliament. Private members' bills do not have a strong record in parliament, but it is not impossible that, if provinces do not act in response to public pressure, Ottawa will.

Summary

Legal and public opinion in Canada appears to weigh heavily against all aspects of *commercial surrogacy*. Where provincial legislation on adoption and child welfare does not explicitly bar surrogate parenting for a fee, it is likely to do so in the future. And the practice would certainly be subject to penalty if federal legislation like Bill C-284 were to be passed. For these and other reasons, there is strong presumption against the practice within Canada in the legal profession. Only in Ontario has regulative permission been proposed, and the report of the Ontario Law Reform Commission has not had widespread support.

We urge that, notwithstanding the real pain of infertility, society put its resources into other cures and couples examine their need or right to have children by almost any means, rather than resorting to a practice which Canadian legal tradition seems to have properly resisted: the casual (and certainly the paid) transfer of parenting away from the birth mother.

We urge those who agree with our findings to participate in the clarification and passage of provincial and federal laws which would ban surrogate parenting on a commercial basis and discourage its practice generally.

We call upon all Canadians to consider the matter of surrogate parenting with a view to minimizing the serious risks it poses to women who are vulnerable to commercial exploitation, to the self-identity of children, and to the integrity of family life which should not be broken in order to "help" another family.

Notes

1. The uncertainties arising from the recent decision of the Supreme Court to strike down previous federal legislation on abortion is a poignant case in point. For an interesting discussion on the general issues of law, morality, and religion *see* Patrick Devlin, *The Enforcement of Morals* (Oxford: Oxford University Press, 1965).
2. A 1986 New York state court ruling, for example, "upheld the payment of money in connection with [a] surrogacy arrangement on the ground that the New York Legislature did not contemplate surrogacy when the baby selling statute was passed. . . . Despite the court's ethical and moral problems with surrogate arrangements, it concluded that the Legislature was the appropriate forum to address the legality of surrogacy arrangements." (Cited in the September 1987 finding of the Supreme Court of New Jersey judgment on the now famous case of Baby M.) As we will show later, very few U.S. state legislatures have yet passed legislation on the matter.

3. The New York State Task Force on Life and the Law, *Surrogate Parenting: Analysis and Recommendations for Public Policy* (May 1988), p. 97.
4. Another useful summary of international studies of an official or quasi-official nature is that of LeRoy Walters, "Ethics and the New Reproductive Technologies," *Hastings Center Report*, June 1987, pp. 3-9.
5. *Report of the Committee of Inquiry into Human Fertilisation and Embryology* (London: H.M. Stationery Office, 1984). A useful summary is to be found in Diana Brahams, "The Hasty British Ban on Commercial Surrogacy," *Hastings Center Report*, February 1987, pp. 16-19.
6. Brahams, "The Hasty British Ban," p. 17.
7. Australian studies frequently cited are those of the Victoria Committee to Consider the Social, Ethical and Legal Issues Arising from In Vitro Fertilization; it is commonly referred to as the Waller Committee.
8. See the analysis by Peter Singer, "Making laws on babies," *Hastings Center Report*, August 1985, pp. 5-6.
9. New York State Task Force report, p. 99.
10. New York State Task Force report, Appendix A, p. 3.
11. Ontario Law Reform Commission, *Report on Human Artificial Reproduction and Related Matters* (1985), Vol. I, p. 91.
12. In a very real sense surrogate parenting is an old rather than a new story. Couples or, more commonly, men have "solved" the problem of female infertility by going outside the marital relationship to "get children" by other women — slaves, second wives, mistresses — for centuries; and there is little reason to think the practice will stop soon without a change in attitudes toward the perceived "need" or "right" to parent. Thus surrogate parenting is controversial because it is simply a new twist on an ancient practice which many find repugnant as an abuse of women and a distortion of parenting as a blessing rather than a right. But for further reflections on this, see other parts of this report.
13. O.L.R.C. report, p. 91. The "rebuttability" refers to the fatherhood of the child. That is, the genetic father may attempt to establish paternity, but it is a *prima facie* presumption that, in law as well as "by nature," as it were, the birthing mother is the legal mother.
14. Children's Law Reform Act (Ontario), section 1 (1).
15. O.L.R.C. report, p. 92.
16. O.L.R.C. report, p. 93.

17. "*Contracts* to transfer custody were declared to be void as against public policy and unenforceable." O.L.R.C. report, p. 92, our italics. The reference is to very early cases, but the principle of declaring void and unenforceable contracts which are "against public policy" is what persists in common law understanding generally, and this principle is frequently used in the matter of surrogate parenting.
18. O.L.R.C. report, p. 95.
19. O.L.R.C. report, p. 100.
20. In Ontario this is covered by section 67 of the Child Welfare Act.
21. O.L.R.C. report, p. 101.
22. O.L.R.C. report, pp. 281-84 (our italics).
23. Barreau du Québec, *Les enjeux éthiques et juridiques des nouvelles technologies de reproduction* (avril 1988).

Conclusions and Recommendations

General Conclusions

Our discussions have led us to a number of conclusions. We identified principles that we think important to uphold, and some recommendations that might be directed to General Synod, to provincial and federal legislators, to infertile couples, to women who are considering acting as a birth mother for them, to medical practitioners, lawyers and pastoral counsellors, to parish study groups, and to any other interested and concerned persons.

Language

We must be careful in the use of language. In discussing surrogacy arrangements it must be clear that the woman who bears a child is the mother of the child. She is not a surrogate in any way. The surrogacy involved when by contract children are conceived and born for others applies to the woman who adopts and raises the child in place of the one who gives birth. To refer to the woman who gives birth to a child as a "surrogate" obscures the actual relationship of the natural birth mother to the child.

Surrogacy and Human Dignity

Human beings must be treated as ends, not means. The humanity of women must not be subordinated to their reproductive capacities. Nor may children be deliberately created for sale. These two grave ethical flaws are inherent in surrogate motherhood. The buying and selling of human beings, for whatever purpose, incorporates the evil present in slavery and is just as offensive. The acquisition of children through payment reduces them to a market commodity. The worth of a human being is not defined by exchange value. We reject a value system that promotes the commodification of persons and their relationships. The human dignity of a child is violated when he or she is treated as an object of sale. No one has an inviolable right to have a child. Nor does anyone have the right to acquire a child by any means, even in the unfortunate event of infertility. Parenthood must be freely

Womanhood

For women, womanhood is to be accepted as synonymous with personhood, not motherhood. A woman is a full human being, and the attitudes that completely identify womanhood with motherhood undermine her aspirations to full human life. Parenthood is obviously a very important part of many women's lives, but it is not the whole of their life. A woman is a human being prior to any activity or role she assumes. We are glad we live in a time when women at long last are beginning to assert that their identity as full persons is not defined by their sexuality and biological capacity. The fulfilment which bearing and caring for children can bring must be seen in the full dimensions of life and the varied needs to which women's diverse gifts can be creatively dedicated. A woman who desires but cannot conceive and bear a child is no less a human being than any other.

The inadequacy and perhaps inferiority that many women feel in not being physically able to have children is in part a social and ecclesiastical responsibility: society and the church have identified motherhood as the essence of femininity. In overvaluing motherhood by locating her actualization in her reproductive power, the Christian churches risk imposing an intolerable burden of guilt on a woman who cannot have children. Christians must rethink their images of women and their attitudes toward them in order to affirm their full humanity as not contingent upon maternity.

We must be vigilant to avoid the abuse of women. The woman who raises the child of her husband and another woman under a contract baby arrangement is in danger of marginalization. She may feel compelled to consent to her husband's contracting with another woman for "his" child as compensation for "her" inadequacy.

Marriage and Fertility

Christians affirm the sanctity and integrity of marriage. Within this understanding, infertility is the condition of a couple, not of one person within the couple. The church upholds the unitive value of marriage as an end in itself. The integrity of marriage is rooted in the mutual love and respect between the woman and man and is not inherently undermined by the absence of procreative capacity.

Parenting and Fatherhood
Paternity may be reduced to a merely genetic connection, but parenting requires the commitment to love and raise a child according to the best of one's abilities. It is a social and interpersonal relationship. A man deserves respect as a father by virtue of his commitment as a parent and not because of the presence of his genes in the child. A man who enters into a contractual arrangement in order to realize his biological paternity may be subordinating both the resulting child and his wife to an ill-understood desire to reproduce his physical self.

Wholeness
As a faith community seeking fullness of life for all, the Christian church places high value on the wholeness for which human beings long. It seeks healing and consolation for those in distress. The psychological and emotional pain experienced by couples who want children but are unable to conceive and bear them should not be underestimated. People whose desire to have children remains unfulfilled must be treated with humane understanding and sensitivity by the church. They should be encouraged to affirm the value of their individual and married life without children of their own bodies.

The use of innovative means to remedy human infertility is a natural expression of our human, rational, and personal transcendence over the material and biological. In assessing the merits of these interventions, we need to keep before us the dignity and wholeness of persons. When thinking about solutions to infertility the primary focus must be on women and children, on their humanity and dignity, and on protection of their interests, as well as on the integrity of the marriage relationship.

Towards a Social Consensus

We call for wide discussion about the values and meanings of personhood and relationships in today's society. The question of surrogacy will be answered in the existing social context. That context needs to be examined and transformed as we move towards a social consensus. The church must take part in the critique, including a critique of its own teaching, structures, and behaviour. To what extent do we as Christians contribute to the destructive, and to what extent to the creative elements in this context?

Stereotypes and Limits

There are many questions to be asked in this discussion. How can we change the attitudes which make it difficult for a woman to feel that her womanhood is complete without the experience of motherhood? If a childless marriage is seen by some to be flawed, what will help a childless couple to value their relationship and celebrate its creativity? How can society encourage a realistic acceptance of the limits of the human condition, and avoid the individualistic presumption that there is a right to free access to all technological possibilities without consideration of the wider social context? Under what conditions is society prepared to impose its own limits? How do we avoid the view that because something can be done it should be permissible? We agree with an observation about surrogacy made by the New York State Task Force on Life and the Law: "Advances in genetic engineering and the cloning and freezing of gametes may soon offer an array of new social options and potential commercial opportunities. An arrangement that transforms human reproductive capacity into a commodity is therefore especially problematic at the present time." How can our society be encouraged to draw the line here?

Humane Responses

As a humane response to those for whom infertility causes personal anguish, more research into the causes of infertility, more education to prevent and reduce its incidence, and more services to ensure its early detection and treatment are all needed. In the allocation of public funds such research, education, and services should be given a higher priority. Quite apart from the serious ethical difficulties concerning the use of human embryos, the heavy investment of resources in programs for *in vitro* fertilization, which in any case have a low success rate, seems hard to justify.

People rightly react with revulsion to crude notions of buying babies or renting wombs. How can we articulate and celebrate the positive ideals implicit in their revulsion, such as those related to whole personhood experienced in healthy relationships?

How can people be helped to see the power structures and dynamics in our male-dominated society, in which women still do not enjoy full equality and still are socialized to regard childbirth as their ultimate fulfilment and social role? What steps can be taken to expose the real risk of exploitation of women even in unpaid and altruistic "surrogate" motherhood?

Surrogacy: A False Solution
There may be people who agree in general with some or all of our arguments against surrogacy but who consider their circumstances unique. Infertile couples, women who are considering acting as a birth mother for them, medical practitioners, lawyers, and pastoral counsellors are understandably inclined to give weight to special pleading. But there is an important and often overlooked point: surrogacy is not a new technology to solve a unique problem. It is essentially a social arrangement by which a family is "built" for infertile couples at the inevitable cost of severing the mother-child bond and thus destroying another family structure. It is highly questionable whether the social order can justify such a practice as a balance of good and evil, especially in light of the potential for abuse in surrogacy. The widely publicized case of Baby M was one in which the adopting mother was not, in fact, infertile; other "special circumstances" can easily be imagined. Legislation to prevent abuses while legitimating and regulating surrogacy, in our view, is the wrong approach; even without abuse, one family bond is created by destroying another. We believe the social arrangement which surrogacy is should be strongly discouraged as "not in the interest of the social order." There are other ways of dealing with infertility which do not carry the same socially destructive impact.

Recommendations on Legal Aspects

1. We endorse the view, which we understand is embedded in common and statute law in Canada, that a woman who gives birth to a child is the child's "natural," and hence legal,

mother. We therefore believe that the terms *natural mother* or *birth mother*, rather than *surrogate mother*, should be employed in any legislation on surrogacy arrangements.
2. We believe that any agreement or contract between a birth mother and others to surrender her care and custody of a child, other than agreements freely entered into after the birth and in the context of adoption law, should be void and unenforceable. To this end we encourage provincial legislators to review and revise adoption laws accordingly, if necessary.
3. In particular, we urge that provincial adoption laws be refined and standardized to ensure that: 1) no payment of money may be promised or made for such adoption, ii) irrevocable adoption occurs only after the birth of a child and an appropriate period of time for the mother to reconsider her decision, and iii) the overriding interest be the best interests of the child, i.e., no preferential option be given to the genetic father (and/or the genetic mother, if pregnancy occurs by embryo transfer) which would override the child's best interests.
4. If provincial adoption laws cannot ensure that commercial surrogacy is banned in Canada, we recommend that federal legislation be enacted making it a criminal offence to recommend, initiate, arrange, or agree to the bearing of a child in a surrogacy arrangement for payment in cash or kind.
5. We further recommend that studies be undertaken to investigate ways in which international law might be enacted and enforced to ensure that Canadians do not use legal loopholes in other countries in order to engage in commercial surrogacy arrangements.
6. None of these recommendations should be implemented in such a way as to violate the principle that a mother may properly wish to serve the long-range best interests of the child to whom she gives birth by placing her/him into the care of others by properly sanctioned adoption procedures.

Proposed Resolutions for General Synod

Resolution A
Be it resolved that this General Synod of the Anglican Church of Canada:

1. Accept the report of the Task Force on "Surrogate Motherhood" for publication and;
2. Commmend it to the church and community for study and action.

Resolution B
Be it resolved that this General Synod of the Anglican Church of Canada agrees that:

1. We affirm the meaning of Christian marriage to be a full and complete sacrament of the unity between two persons in and of itself. We support those who have entered into this covenant.
2. We understand that the procreation of children is a good that might come out of a couple's mutual love, but the absence of children in no way renders a marriage incomplete.
3. We affirm any married couple's desire for children from their union. But we ask all couples, their friends and families, to consider the reality of various limitations, for example, fertility, personality, or genetic impairment, which may make children for them either impossible, hurtful, or simply unwise. We ask our Christian communities to uphold those who are living within such limitations or restrictions.
4. We find the practice of "surrogate motherhood" to be an unacceptable means of acquiring children, whether undertaken as a financial or charitable transaction. We find that this dehumanizing practice reduces human life in the "image of God" to a commodity. It removes the creation of new life from the sacramental relationship of woman and man in mutual love. It leaves a legacy for both birth mother and child which in all likelihood will be hurtful and destructive.
5. We express our ethical concern that the practice of "surrogate motherhood" will abuse women by denying their role as the actual bearers and mothers of children.
6. We pledge our support to couples who would wish to have children from their union but find themselves unable to do so. We pray that they will find satisfaction for this longing without resorting to any technology or practice which may ultimately be disrespectful or destructive to them, their marriage,

a child, or any other person. We encourage technologies and practices which do respect each of these.

Resolution C
Be it resolved that this General Synod of the Anglican Church of Canada urge:

1. That as a matter of public policy surrogate parenting should be discouraged,
2. That surrogacy contracts should be unenforceable in Canada,
3. That the recommendations on legal aspects concerned in the report (page 8) (see pages 97-98) be endorsed,
4. That the principles and recommendations in the report of the Task Force on "Surrogate Motherhood" together with the resolutions of this 32nd General Synod of the Anglican Church of Canada which relate to surrogacy be the basis of any recommendations by the National Executive Council and other national church bodies to governments when policy is being formed or legislation enacted, and
5. That the above resources be commended also to the provinces and dioceses of the Anglican Church of Canada.

Members of an Anglican Task Force on "Surrogate Motherhood"

The Right Reverend J.A. Baycroft, M.A., D.D.
Suffragan Bishop of the Anglican Diocese of Ottawa, Chair

The Reverend Professor Bruce Alton, Ph.D.,
Trinity College, Toronto

Phyllis Creighton, M.A.,
Historian, Researcher, Editor, University of Toronto Press

Professor Marsha Hewitt, Ph.D.,
Trinity College, Toronto

The Reverend Professor Don Thompson, Ph.D.,
Centre for Christian Studies, Toronto

Response of Synod

In June 1989 the General Synod of the Anglican Church of Canada, meeting in St. John's, Newfoundland, passed three resolutions based on the report of a Task Force on "Surrogate Motherhood." The official resolutions of General Synod are:

Surrogate Motherhood

Act 70
That the report of the Task Force on "Surrogate Motherhood" be:

a) accepted for publication: and
b) commended to the Church and community for study and action.

Surrogacy and Christian Marriage

Act 71
That this General Synod of the Anglican Church of Canada agree that:

1. We affirm marriage, as a lifelong union in faithful love to the exclusion of all others on either side, to be a full and complete sacrament of the unity between two persons in and of itself. We support those who have entered into this covenant.
2. We understand that the procreation of children is a good that might come out of a couple's mutual love, but the absence of children in itself does not compromise the integrity and value of a marriage.
3. We affirm any married couple's desire for children from their union. But we ask all couples, their friends and families, to consider the reality of various limitations for example, fertility, personality, or genetic impairment which may make children for them either impossible, hurtful or simply unwise. We ask our Christian communities to uphold those who are living within such limitations or restrictions.

4. We find the practice of "surrogate motherhood" to be an unacceptable means of acquiring children, whether undertaken as a financial or charitable transaction. We find that this dehumanizing practice reduces human life in the new "image of God" to a commodity. It removes the creation of new life from the sacramental relationship of woman and man in mutual love. It leaves a legacy for both birth mother and child which in all likelihood will be hurtful and destructive.
5. We express our ethical concern that the practice of "surrogate motherhood" will abuse women by denying their role as the actual bearers and mothers of children.
6. We pledge our support to couples who would wish to have children from their union but find themselves unable to do so. We pray that they will find satisfaction for this longing without resorting to any technology or practice which may ultimately be disrespectful or destructive to them, their marriage, a child, or any other person. We encourage technologies and practices which do respect each of these.
7. We affirm adoptive parents and adopted children in the life of the church as full members of the Christian family.

Surrogate Parenting

Act 112

That this General Synod of the Anglican Church of Canada:

1. Urge that as a matter of public policy surrogate parenting should be discouraged.
2. Urge that surrogacy contracts should be unenforceable in Canada.
3. Adopt recommendations 1, 2, 3, 5 and 6 on legal aspects contained in the report of the Anglican Task Force on Surrogate Motherhood on pages 8 and 9. (See pages 97 and 98 of this report.)
4. Recommend to the provinces and territories that adoption laws ensure that commercial surrogacy (recommending, initiating, arranging, or agreeing to the bearing of a child in a surrogacy arrangement for payment in cash or in kind) is banned in each province and territory.

5. Agree that the principles and recommendations in the report of the Task Force on "Surrogate Motherhood", together with the resolutions of this 32nd General Synod of the Anglican Church of Canada which relate to surrogacy be the basis of any recommendations by the National Executive Council and other national Church bodies to governments when policy is being formed or legislation enacted.
6. Commend the above resources also to the Provinces and Dioceses of the Anglican Church of Canada.

These resolutions express the mind of the Anglican Church of Canada as discerned by the General Synod. The report is published on the authority of Act 70, but, as will be seen by comparing, for example, Act 112 with the recommendations on legal aspects on page 9, (see pages 97 and 98 of this report) General Synod did not feel obliged to agree with every detail of what the task force suggested. However, the discussion stimulated by the report and the overwhelming support by General Synod for the basic position taken by the task force encourage us to believe that both the official resolutions and this report as a whole will contribute to the continuing discussion of the serious issues identified here.

John Baycroft
Chair of an Anglican Task Force
on "Surrogate Motherhood"

Appendix

Executive Summary

From *Surrogate Parenting: Analysis and Recommendations for Public Policy*, The New York State Task Force on Life and the Law, May 1988

The Task Force's conclusions and recommendations regarding surrogate parenting are summarized below. The recommendations have the unanimous support of the Task Force membership. The Task Force has developed a legislative proposal that appears as an appendix to this Report.

Part I: The Medical, Legal and Social Context

Surrogate parenting is not a technology, but a social arrangement that uses reproductive technology (usually artificial insemination) to enable one woman to produce a child for a man and, if he is married, for his wife. Surrogate parenting is characterized by the intention to separate the genetic and/or gestational aspects of child bearing from parental rights and responsibilities through an agreement to transfer the infant and maternal rights at birth.

The well-publicized Baby M case has given surrogate parenting a prominent place on the public agenda. Nonetheless, the reproductive technologies used in the arrangements — artificial insemination and, increasingly, in vitro fertilization — also pose profound questions about the ethical, social and biological bases of parenthood. In addition, the procedures to screen donors raise important public health concerns. The Task Force will address these issues in its ongoing deliberations and recognizes that they form part of the context within which surrogate parenting must be considered.

Legal questions about surrogate parenting, although novel in many respects, arise within the framework of a well-developed body of New York family law. In particular, policies about surrogate parenting will necessarily focus upon two basic concerns in all matters involving the care and custody of children — the protection of the fundamental right of a parent to rear his or her child and the promotion of the child's best interests.

The Supreme Court of New Jersey has ruled that paying a surrogate violates state laws against baby selling. Surrogacy agreements may also be found invalid because they conflict with comprehensive statutory schemes that govern private adoption and the termination of parental rights.

In New York, it is uncertain whether surrogate parenting contracts are barred by the statute that prohibits payments for adoption. If not, it is probable that the surrogate could transfer the child to the intended parents by following private adoption procedures. If a dispute about parental rights arises before the surrogate consents to the child's adoption, custody would probably be determined based on the child's best interests. Regardless of the outcome, the court ordinarily will have no basis for terminating the parental status of either the surrogate or the intended father.

The right to enter into and enforce surrogate parenting arrangements is not protected as part of the constitutional right to privacy. Surrogate parenting involves social and contractual — rather than individual — decisions and arrangements that may place the rights and interests of several individuals in direct conflict. The commercial aspects of surrogate parenting also distinguish the practice from other constitutionally protected private acts. Constitutional protection for the right to privacy is diminished when the conduct involved assumes a commercial character.

The social and moral issues posed by surrogate parenting touch upon five central concerns (i) individual access and social responsibility in the face of new reproductive possibilities; (ii) the interests of children; (iii) the impact of the practice on family life and relationships; (iv) attitudes about reproduction and women; and (v) application of the informed consent doctrine.

Surrogate parenting has been the subject of extensive scrutiny by public and private groups, including governmental bodies in the United States and abroad, religious communities, professional organizations, women's rights organizations and groups that advocate on behalf of children and infertile couples. Of the governmental commissions that have studied the issue, many concluded that surrogate parenting is unacceptable. In this country, six states have enacted laws on surrogate parenting, four of which declare surrogate contracts void and unenforceable as against public policy.

Part II: Deliberations and Recommendations of the Task Force
As evidenced by the large body of statutory law on custody and adoption, society has a basic interest in protecting the best interests of children and in shielding gestation and reproduction from the flow of commerce.

When surrogate parenting involves the payment of fees and a contractual obligation to relinquish the child at birth, it places children at risk and is not in their best interests. The practice also has the potential to undermine the dignity of women, children and human reproduction.

Surrogate parenting alters deep-rooted social and moral assumptions about the relationship between parents and their children. The practice involves unprecedented rules and standards for terminating parental obligations and rights, including the right to a relationship with one's own child. The assumption that "a deal is a deal," relied upon to justify this drastic change in public policy, fails to respect the significance of the relationships and rights at stake.

Advances in genetic engineering and the cloning and freezing of gametes may soon offer an array of new social options and potential commercial opportunities. An arrangement that transforms human reproductive capacity into a commodity is therefore especially problematic at the present time.

Public policy should discourage surrogate parenting. This goal should be achieved through legislation that declares the contracts void as against public policy. In addition, legislation should prohibit fees for surrogates and bar surrogate brokers from operating in New York State. These measures are designed to eliminate commercial surrogacy and the growth of a business community or industry devoted to making money from human reproduction and the birth of children.

The legislation proposed by the Task Force would not prohibit surrogate parenting arrangements when they are not commercial and remain undisputed. Existing law permits each stage of the arrangement under these circumstances; a decision by a woman to be artificially inseminated or to have an embryo implanted; her voluntary decision after the child's birth to relinquish the child for adoption; and the child's adoption by the intended parents.

Under existing law on adoption, the intended parents would be permitted to pay reasonable expenses associated with pregnancy and childbirth to a mother who relinquishes her child for adoption. All such expenses must be approved by a court as part of an adoption proceeding.

In custody disputes arising from surrogate parenting arrangements, the birth mother and her husband, if any, should be awarded custody unless the court finds, based on clear and convincing evidence, that the child's best interests would be served by an award of custody to the father and/or genetic mother. The court should award visitation and support obligations as it would under existing law in proceedings on these matters.

To date, few programs have been conducted by the public or the private sector to prevent infertility. Programs to educate the public and health care professionals about the causes of infertility and the measures available for early detection and treatment could spare many couples from facing the problem. Both the government and the medical community should establish educational and other programs to prevent infertility. Resources should also be devoted to research about the causes and nature of infertility.